Core Exercises for Seniors

Strengthen Your Body and Improve Balance with Easy-to-Follow Step-by-Step Instructions

Free Bonuses from Scott Hamrick

Hi seniors!

My name is Scott Hamrick, and first off, I want to THANK YOU for reading my book.

Now you have a chance to join my exclusive "workout for seniors" email list so you can get the ebook below for free as well as the potential to get more ebooks for seniors for free! Simply click the link below to join.

P.S. Remember that it's 100% free to join the list.

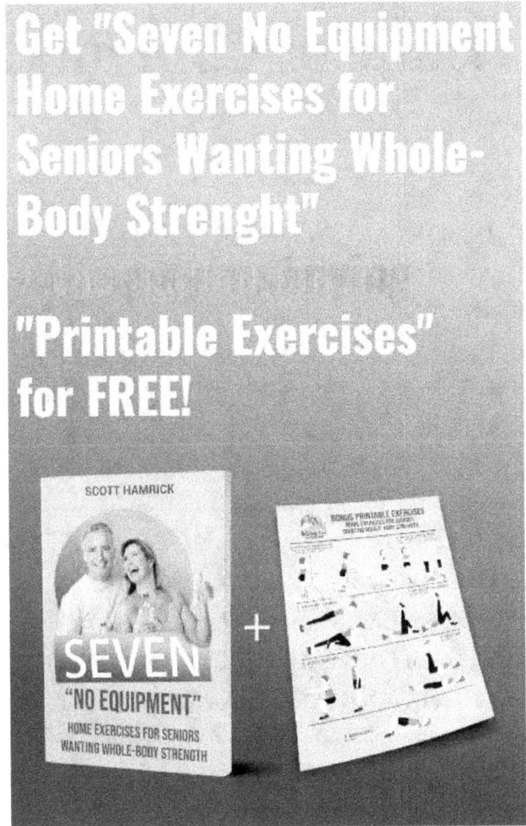

Access your free bonuses here
https://livetolearn.lpages.co/core-exercises-for-seniors-paperback/

Table of Contents

Introduction

As we grow older, keeping our core strength and stability becomes increasingly important. Statistics show that maintaining a strong core can significantly enhance our quality of life in our senior years. Research indicates that individuals with a strong core are 25% less likely to experience injuries related to falls, such as fractures and sprains. Moreover, it can lead to a 30% reduction in the risk of developing poor posture, which can contribute to back pain and discomfort.

Engaging in simple core exercises can make a big difference. Studies reveal that just 15 minutes of core-focused workouts three times a week can improve balance by 20%. This translates into greater confidence when navigating everyday tasks like bending over to tie your shoes or lifting groceries from the car.

In essence, a strong core isn't just about looking good; it's about enjoying a happier, healthier senior life. By dedicating a small amount of time to core-strengthening exercises, you can significantly enhance your overall well-being, reduce the risk of falls, and maintain your independence as you age.

What sets "Core Exercises for Seniors" apart from the rest? It's all about simplicity and hands-on methods. We understand that complex workouts can be intimidating and discouraging. That's why our book is designed with clear, step-by-step instructions that anyone can follow.

Whether you're a complete beginner or someone who's been out of the fitness game for a while, our book is your perfect companion. We break down each exercise into easy-to-follow movements, ensuring you can start at your own pace and gradually build up your strength. You'll never feel overwhelmed or lost on your fitness journey.

What can you expect from "Core Exercises for Seniors"? First and foremost, you'll discover a collection of core exercises that are tailored specifically for seniors. No more sifting through generic fitness routines that may not suit your needs. Our book is laser-focused on what matters most to you.

But it's not just about the exercises. We provide you with valuable insights into the benefits of core strength, helping you understand why it's so essential for your well-being. You'll learn how these exercises can alleviate back pain, boost your energy levels, and enhance your overall quality of life.

Additionally, we've included modifications and variations for each exercise, ensuring that you can tailor your workouts to your individual needs and capabilities. No matter your fitness level or any physical limitations you may have, you'll find a suitable exercise routine within these pages.

Are you ready to take the first step toward a healthier, more vibrant you? "Core Exercises for Seniors" is a book that will guide you every step of the way. With its easy-to-understand instructions, beginner-friendly approach, and hands-on methods, you'll feel inspired and motivated to start your fitness journey today.

Don't wait any longer to improve your balance, strengthen your body, and enjoy a more active lifestyle. Join countless seniors who have already transformed their lives with the power of core exercises. Your path to better health begins here – in the pages of our book. Start reading now and take the first step toward a happier, healthier you!

Chapter 1: The Importance of the Core

The core is more than just a set of muscles; it's the powerhouse of your body. To age gracefully, you need to understand its importance. Picture this: the core is like the sturdy foundation of a building. Without it, everything else crumbles. In this chapter, we will explore the core's anatomy and unravel its vital role in everyday life!

At its core (pun intended), the core comprises several muscles, primarily the rectus abdominis, obliques, and the transverse abdominis. These muscles wrap around your midsection like a protective shield. But they do more than give you those coveted six-pack abs. These muscles are the unsung heroes behind every move you make.

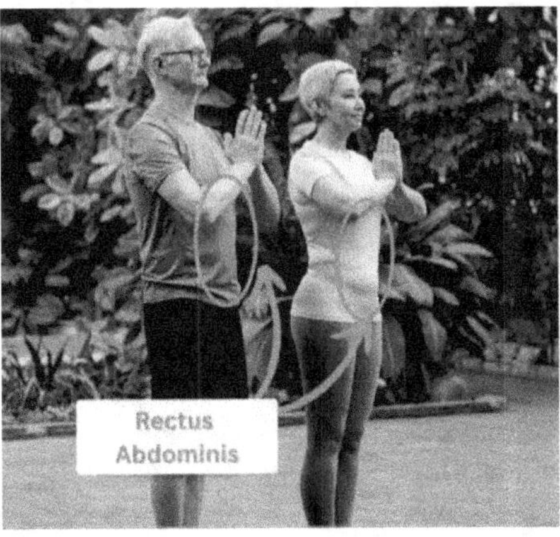

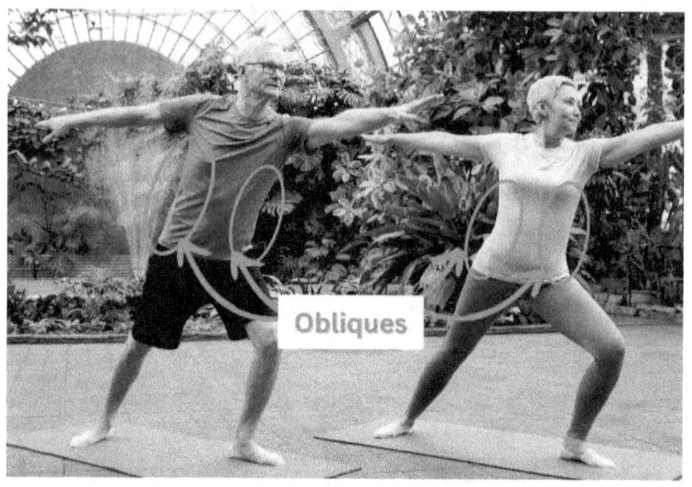

https://www.pexels.com/photo/couple-practicing-yoga-6787440/

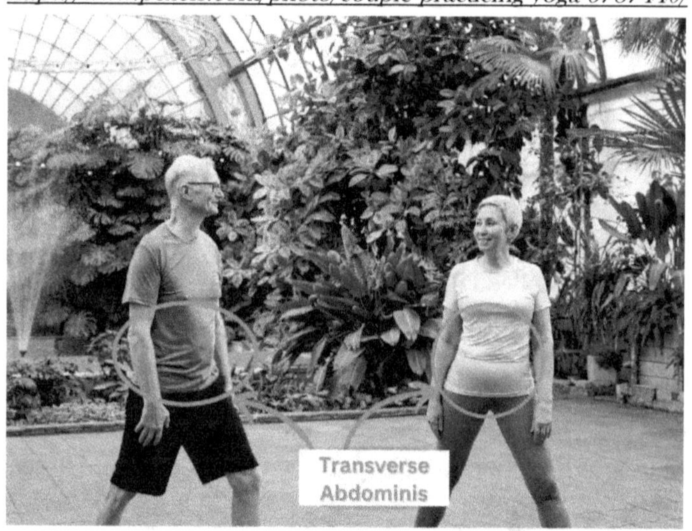

https://www.pexels.com/photo/couple-practicing-yoga-6787501/

But why should you care about these internal workings? Well, here's the secret: your core isn't just about having a beach-ready body. It's about functionality, stability, and overall well-being.

Think about your daily routine. From the moment you get out of bed to reaching for that cup of morning coffee, your core is silently working its magic. When you bend over to tie your shoelaces, your core muscles engage to support your spine and prevent strain. When you reach for a book on a high shelf, your core helps you maintain balance. Every step, every movement, every twist – your core is there, quietly ensuring you can tackle life's challenges with grace.

Imagine picking up a bag of groceries. Your core muscles swing into action, stabilizing your spine and preventing you from toppling over like a Jenga tower. They're like your body's personal bodyguards, protecting your back from injury.

Now, think about balance. Balancing on one foot while tying your shoelaces? Your core muscles are working their magic to keep you upright. They're the tightrope walkers of your body, ensuring you don't stumble and fall.

But it doesn't stop there. Your core is your body's shock absorber. When you take a step, jump, or even laugh, it dampens the impact on your spine, sparing you from a world of pain. It's like having built-in shock absorbers for your body.

As you age, maintaining a strong core becomes even more critical. Picture yourself in your golden years. You want to remain active, right? Your core is your ally in this battle against time. It keeps you steady on your feet, allowing you to enjoy strolls, dance, and play with your grandkids without fear of losing your balance.

Let's not forget about posture. Ever seen someone with a hunchback? Chances are that their core muscles weren't up to the task. A strong core supports an upright posture, helping you stand tall and confident as the years pass. Goodbye, slouching; hello, elegance!

Now, let's talk about the everyday activities we often take for granted. From getting out of bed to reaching for that jar of peanut butter on the top shelf, your core muscles are hard at work. They provide stability, strength, and mobility, making your daily life smoother and more enjoyable.

As we journey through life, challenges come our way. Whether it's lifting a heavy suitcase or bending to tie your shoes, your core is there to lend a helping hand. It's your dependable partner, ensuring you tackle these tasks with ease and grace.

In a world that's constantly changing, one thing remains certain: the importance of the core in helping you age gracefully. Its muscles are not just for show; they are your body's silent heroes, working tirelessly to keep you strong, stable, and injury-free.

Your core is a central hub, connecting all your body's systems. It's not just about physical strength; it impacts your posture, your breathing, and even your digestion. A weak core can cause you to slouch, leading to a host of problems – like back pain and decreased lung capacity. It can also affect how efficiently your digestive system works, potentially leading to discomfort and poor nutrient absorption.

A weak core is more than just a cosmetic concern; it can affect your overall health and daily life. Your core muscles, including your abdominals, lower back, and pelvis, play a crucial role in stabilizing your body and supporting your spine. According to a study published in the Journal of Physical Therapy Science, 64% of people with poor posture had weak core muscles. This highlights a strong connection between the two. When your core is weak, it can lead to a range of signs and symptoms that may not always be obvious.

One of the most noticeable signs of a weak core is poor posture. If you find yourself slouching or hunching over frequently, it's likely due to insufficient core strength. Weak core muscles can also lead to lower back pain. Your core provides support to your spine, and when it's weak, your back muscles may have to compensate, leading to discomfort or pain. The National Institute of Neurological Disorders and Stroke reports that back pain affects 80% of adults at some point. Poor posture due to a weak core can contribute to this problem.

In addition, core muscles are essential for balance. If you often feel unsteady or have difficulty maintaining your balance, your core strength could be to blame. Balance problems often indicate a weak core, and the numbers back it up. According to the National Institute on Aging, 28.7% of people aged 65 and older experience falls each year, with balance issues being a leading cause.

A strong core stabilizes your body, preventing these tumbles. Moreover, poor balance doesn't discriminate by age. A weak core affects not only older adults but also younger individuals. A study in the Journal of Sports Science & Medicine showed that 68% of athletes with balance problems had weaker core muscles.

Surprisingly, a weak core can even affect your digestion! Weak abdominal muscles might lead to digestive problems, such as constipation, as they play a role in supporting the organs involved in digestion. Firstly, constipation can become a common problem. Weak core muscles make it harder for your abdominal muscles to assist in the natural squeezing motion of your intestines, slowing down the movement of food waste.

Additionally, acid reflux may become more frequent. A weak core can cause poor posture, which in turn can lead to a relaxation of the lower esophageal sphincter, allowing stomach acid to flow back into the esophagus. Statistics show that about 20% of Americans suffer from chronic constipation, and nearly 20-30% experience acid reflux symptoms regularly. These numbers highlight the prevalence of digestive issues in the population.

Sometimes, a weak core can also be life-threatening. Weak core muscles can make you more susceptible to injuries, particularly when engaging in physical activities or sports. It's easier to strain or sprain other muscles if your core can't provide the stability needed for these movements. Statistics show that individuals with underdeveloped core muscles are more likely to get injured during physical activities.

A whopping 62% of all sports-related injuries are linked to poor core strength. That's more than half! When your core can't hold its own, other muscles have to compensate. They get overworked and strained, leading to injuries. Think of it this way: if your core is the quarterback, the rest of your muscles are the offensive line. If the quarterback falters, the whole team suffers.

But here's the good news: you don't need to become a gym rat or a fitness fanatic to reap the benefits of a strong core. Simple, everyday exercises can make a world of difference. Imagine doing a gentle set of leg raises while lying on your back or holding a plank for a few seconds each day. These small efforts can gradually build your core strength and improve your overall well-being.

The importance of the core extends beyond physical health; it has a profound impact on your mental and emotional well-being as well. Your core isn't just those muscles you see on fitness posters; it's a whole squad of muscles deep inside your belly and back. They're like your body's secret agents, working hard to keep you stable and balanced. But they're not just for physical stuff; they play a crucial role in how you feel inside.

First off, your core muscles are like a bodyguard for your spine. They keep it straight and strong, which can help reduce back pain. And we all know that when your back feels good, your mood tends to follow suit. So, a strong core can be your secret weapon against those nagging aches that bring your spirits down. But the core's superpowers don't stop there.

When you work on those muscles, you're not just strengthening your body; you're boosting your self-confidence too. It's like wearing an invisible superhero cape. You stand tall and feel more capable, and that positive energy spreads to your mind and emotions. Strengthening your core has a plethora of benefits that can make your daily life better. So, let's dive into the top 10 benefits of having a strong core!

Improved Posture

A strong core helps you stand tall and sit straight. Imagine your core as the anchor of a ship. It keeps everything steady and in the right place. One of its main jobs is to support your spine, that long, bony structure that runs from your neck all the way down to your lower back. When your core is strong, it acts like a reliable bodyguard for your spine, keeping it safe and sound.

Now, let's talk about slouching. We've all been guilty of it at some point – that lazy, hunched-over posture that creeps in when we're tired or not paying attention. But guess what? A strong core is like your body's personal bodyguard against slouching. It stands guard and says, "Nope, not on my watch!" It keeps you upright and prevents the dreaded slouch.

But here's the real magic: a robust core can save you from the perils of poor posture. You know . . . that constant back pain that nags at you like a persistent mosquito! When your core is in tip-top shape, it acts as a buffer, reducing the risk of those annoying posture-related problems.

Better Balance

Core muscles are essential for stability. Strengthening them enhances your balance, reducing the likelihood of falls or injuries, especially as you age. As we age, our bodies naturally lose some of their stability and balance. That's where core strength training becomes even more essential. It's like giving your body an insurance policy against slips, trips, and falls. By keeping your core strong, you're reducing the risk of accidents that can lead to injuries.

Think of your core muscles as your body's built-in safety net. They protect you from those unexpected moments when you might lose your footing or stumble on uneven terrain. And it's not just about preventing falls – a strong core can also help you perform daily tasks with ease, like bending down to pick up something from the floor or reaching for items on high shelves without losing your balance.

So, don't underestimate the power of your core muscles. Strengthening them is like giving your body a shield against instability. It's a practical and smart way to stay agile and injury-free, no matter what your age.

Enhanced Athletic Performance

Whether you're into sports or just enjoy an occasional run, a strong core helps improve your overall athletic performance. It provides a solid foundation for all movements, from running to lifting weights. Now, let's talk about power and speed. Whether you're sprinting, jumping, or throwing, generating power from your core is essential. A strong core allows you to transfer force effectively, making your movements more explosive and efficient. This is particularly beneficial for athletes aiming to improve their performance in sports like basketball, soccer, or track and field.

Moreover, your core is the link between your upper and lower body. It connects your arms and legs, allowing them to work in harmony. When your core is strong, you can maximize the coordination between these limbs, resulting in smoother and more controlled movements. Imagine the precision required in activities like tennis, golf, or even swimming – a strong core is the secret ingredient to excel in these sports.

Back Pain Relief

A weak core can lead to back pain. But a strong one can alleviate or even prevent it by providing the necessary support to your spine and reducing the strain on your lower back. Imagine if your house had a shaky foundation. It wouldn't be able to withstand the stresses of daily life, and cracks might start to appear in the walls. Similarly, if your core is weak, your spine can't handle the stresses of everyday activities, leading to back pain.

But when you have a robust core, it's like having a solid foundation for your body. It helps distribute the weight of your upper body evenly, reducing the strain on your lower back. This is crucial for preventing back pain and maintaining a healthy spine.

So, if you've been dealing with nagging back pain, don't underestimate the power of a strong core. It's not about having six-pack abs or looking like a bodybuilder. It's about giving your spine the support it needs to keep you pain-free and able to move comfortably. Incorporating core-strengthening exercises into your routine can make a world of difference. Simple activities like planks, bridges, and leg raises can help build those essential core muscles.

Boosted Metabolism

Metabolism is the process your body uses to convert the food you eat into energy. A faster metabolism means your body burns more calories, even when you're at rest. Who wouldn't want that?

So, how does strengthening your core help with metabolism? It's all about the exercises you do. Many core-focused workouts engage multiple muscle groups, not just your core muscles. This is fantastic news for your metabolism because it means you're burning more calories during these exercises.

Think about it this way: when you do a plank, you're not just working your abs. You're also engaging your leg muscles, arm muscles, and even your shoulders. All of this activity increases your heart rate and calorie burn, giving your metabolism a nice little kick.

But it's not just about the calories you burn during your workout. A strong core supports your daily activities, making them more energy-efficient. Whether you're picking up groceries or playing with your kids, a solid core helps you do these tasks with ease, which, in turn, helps you burn more calories throughout the day.

Enhanced Breathing

The way you sit or stand can affect your breathing. If your core is weak and your posture slouchy, your lungs can't fully expand. This means you're not getting as much oxygen as you could with proper posture and a strong core. Your lungs are like balloons; they expand and contract with each breath.

A strong core helps create the necessary space for your lungs to expand fully. This means you can take in more oxygen with each breath, leading to enhanced breathing and improved overall respiratory function.

Proper core engagement improves the efficiency of your breathing. When you breathe, your diaphragm, a dome-shaped muscle beneath your ribcage, contracts and flattens. This movement creates a vacuum in your chest cavity, pulling air into your lungs. A strong core supports the diaphragm's movement, making it easier for you to take deep, efficient breaths.

Your blood carries oxygen to all parts of your body. With enhanced breathing due to a strong core, your blood gets a fresh supply of oxygen with each breath. This means your muscles, brain, and every cell in your body receive the oxygen they need to function optimally.

Injury Prevention

When you have a robust core, it's like having a sturdy foundation for a building. When we talk about injury prevention, we often picture padded helmets or knee braces. However, what many people overlook is the incredible role that your core muscles play in safeguarding your body. They're like your body's natural bodyguards, and they do their job quietly but efficiently.

So, what do these core muscles do? Well, they provide incredible support to your joints and muscles. Think of them as the sturdy pillars holding up a bridge. When your core is strong, it helps distribute the load evenly, reducing the strain on other parts of your body. This means you're less likely to experience those nasty twists and sprains that can put you on the sidelines.

Not only do strong core muscles protect you during physical activities, but they also support your posture in everyday life. Slouching at your desk or hunching over your phone can strain your back and neck, leading to discomfort and potential injuries.

Let's not forget about the back. Back pain is a common complaint, and a weak core is often the culprit. When your core isn't doing its job, your back has to pick up the slack, leading to overuse and pain. Strengthening your core can help alleviate this burden and keep your back happy.

A Flatter Tummy (Yes, Really!)

While it's not all about aesthetics, having a strong core can help tone your abdominal muscles. This can lead to a flatter, more toned tummy – a nice bonus!

Now that you know the fantastic benefits of having a strong core, you're probably wondering how to get one. Fortunately, you don't need fancy equipment or hours at the gym. Simple exercises like planks, bridges, and leg raises can do wonders for your core strength. Just remember to start slowly and gradually increase the intensity to avoid injury.

Consistency is key. Aim to incorporate core-strengthening exercises into your routine at least a few times a week. You'll start to notice the benefits in your daily life, from improved posture to increased energy levels.

Chapter 2: The Anatomy of the Core: More Than Just Abs

When we think of the "core," the first image that often comes to mind is a set of chiseled abs, sculpted to perfection. But the core is so much more than just those coveted six-pack muscles. It's like thinking an iceberg is only its tip - there's a whole lot more beneath the surface. So, let's dive in and discover the real deal about the core!

Your core involves a dynamic team of muscles working together. We're talking about the muscles in your back, sides, and even some deep within. They create a muscular girdle that wraps around your midsection, providing stability, support, and strength. Sure, having toned abs looks great at the beach, but the core's real magic happens behind the scenes:

Abdominals

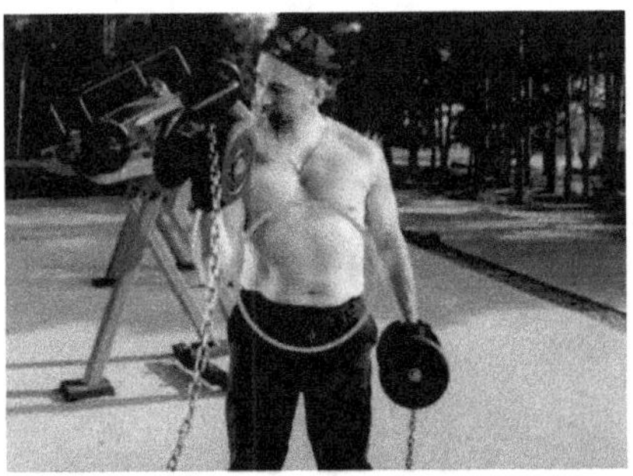

https://www.pexels.com/photo/a-man-lifting-dumbbells-6293106/

The abdominals, often referred to as the abs, are an essential part of your body's core strength. Think of them as your built-in armor, protecting your innermost treasures. These ab muscles are a diverse team, with standout players like the rectus abdominis, known for its distinctive "six-pack" appearance, and the obliques, the dependable sidekicks. Together, they form a powerhouse that does more than meets the eye.

The rectus abdominis is like the showstopper of this team. It's the muscle responsible for the eye-catching six-pack look that many people desire. Located in the front and center of your abdomen, this muscle is the key player in flexing your torso, allowing you to bend forward and sit up. When you're doing crunches or sit-ups, you're giving your rectus abdominis a workout.

But wait, there's more to the story. Your obliques, situated on the sides of your abdomen, are equally crucial. They come in two types: the internal and external obliques. These muscles allow you to twist and turn your torso, giving you the agility to reach for something behind you or swing a golf club with precision.

Now, let's talk about protection. Your abdominals serve as a natural shield for your vital organs. Just beneath that six-pack or those obliques, your liver, intestines, and other precious internal organs find sanctuary. These muscles act as a barrier, cushioning your innards from potential harm. It's like having a personal bodyguard for your organs.

Back Muscles

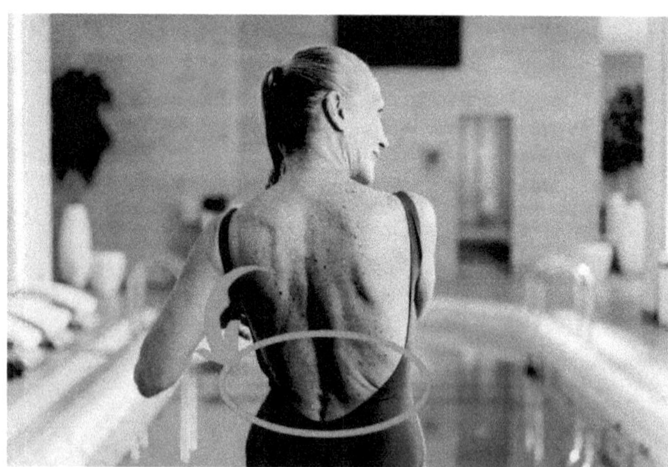

Back muscles play a crucial role in supporting your spine and facilitating various upper-body movements. Think of them as the strong ropes that hold up a sturdy tent, ensuring stability and functionality. In this article, we will delve deeper into the fascinating world of back muscles, specifically focusing on the erector spinae and latissimus dorsi.

The erector spinae, located on either side of your spine, are essential for maintaining an upright posture. Comprising three muscle groups – the iliocostalis, longissimus, and spinalis – these muscles work harmoniously to keep your spine straight. When you stand or sit upright, it's your erector spinae that prevents you from slouching and supports your vertebral column. They are the unsung heroes behind your effortless posture.

Additionally, the erector spinae muscles are instrumental in controlling the motion of your spine. Whether you're bending forward to pick up an object or arching backward to stretch, these muscles are actively engaged. They provide the necessary stability and control for these movements, preventing any potential injuries to your spine.

Now, let's turn our attention to the latissimus dorsi, often referred to as the "lats." These large, fan-shaped muscles are situated on your back's sides, resembling mighty wings. While they may not help you fly, they play a pivotal role in various upper-body movements.

The primary function of the latissimus dorsi is to perform shoulder extension, which involves pulling your arm downward and backward. This action is especially evident when you perform exercises like pull-ups or rowing, where your lats are heavily engaged. They give you the strength to perform these movements with ease and efficiency.

Moreover, the latissimus dorsi also contributes to shoulder adduction, which is the act of bringing your arm closer to your body's midline. This function is essential for movements such as reaching across your body or performing a strong, controlled swim stroke.

In essence, your back muscles, including the erector spinae and latissimus dorsi, are not just passive support structures. They are dynamic and powerful, enabling you to maintain an upright posture, perform everyday activities, and engage in various forms of exercise.

Pelvic Floor

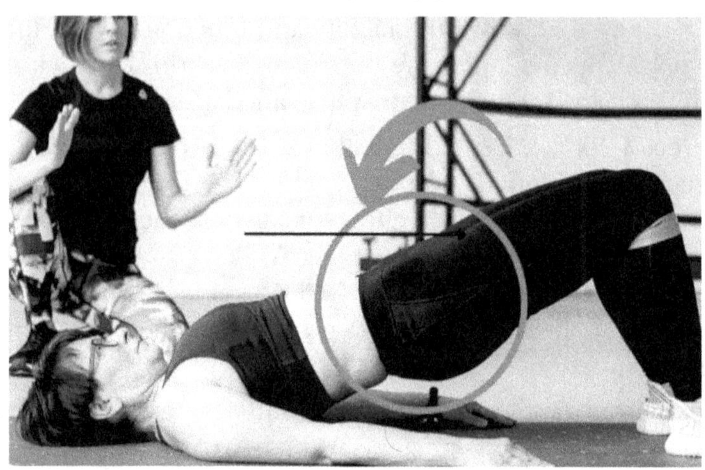

Imagine your pelvic floor as a trusty trampoline beneath you. This remarkable group of muscles, tucked away at the base of your spine, plays a crucial role in supporting and safeguarding your pelvic organs, such as your bladder and intestines. Understanding the importance of your pelvic floor can help you maintain stability and control over your body.

The pelvic floor may not be a topic that often comes up in daily conversations, but it deserves our attention. These muscles form a strong and flexible foundation that acts like a hammock, cradling your pelvic organs and ensuring they stay in their proper places. Without this support system, daily activities like standing, sitting, or even sneezing would be much more challenging.

Your pelvic floor is a complex web of muscles, ligaments, and connective tissues. It resembles a woven basket, with various muscle groups working together harmoniously. These muscles are responsible for maintaining the position and functioning of your pelvic organs.

Think about your bladder, which holds urine, and your intestines, responsible for digestion. These organs need a reliable support system to function correctly. Your pelvic floor steps up to the plate, ensuring they remain in place and operate smoothly.

When your pelvic floor muscles are strong and healthy, they provide the necessary support to keep your bladder and intestines from sagging or bulging into the vagina or rectum. This prevents issues like urinary incontinence and pelvic organ prolapse, conditions that can significantly impact your quality of life.

Your pelvic floor isn't just about support; it's also crucial for stability and control. These muscles work in harmony with your core muscles, helping you maintain proper posture and balance. When you engage your pelvic floor, it contributes to a strong and stable core, which is essential for various physical activities.

Diaphragm

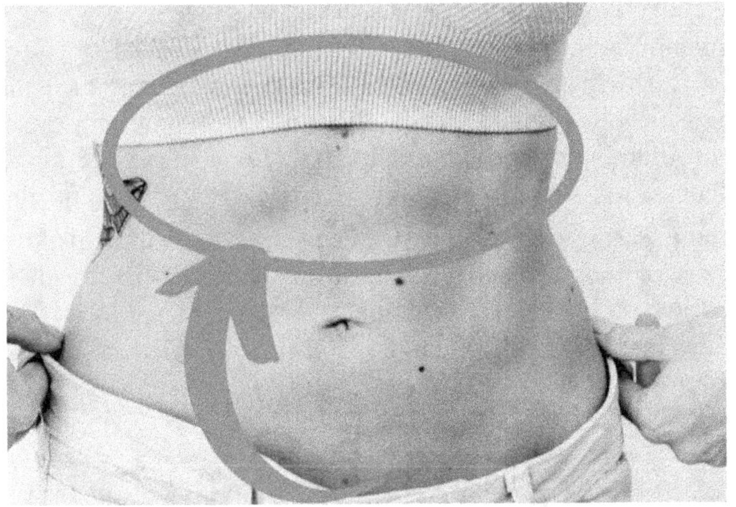

Located just beneath your lungs, the diaphragm is a marvel of nature. Its unique dome-shaped structure is designed for efficiency. When you inhale, this powerful muscle contracts, flattening out like a parachute deploying. This action creates a vacuum in your chest, drawing air into your lungs effortlessly. Exhaling, on the other hand, is a relaxing moment for the diaphragm as it returns to its dome shape, pushing air out.

But the diaphragm is not just about breathing; it's a multi-tasker. When you lift heavy objects or engage in strenuous activities, your diaphragm becomes your steadfast ally. It plays a crucial role in stabilizing your core and protecting your spine. Think of it as the strong anchor that prevents you from wobbling when you pick up that hefty box or perform a strenuous exercise.

Moreover, the diaphragm is a team player. It collaborates with your abdominal muscles, forming a dynamic duo that provides essential support for your lower back. Together, they maintain proper posture and reduce the risk of injury. So, next time you bend over to tie your shoes or deadlift at the gym, remember to thank your diaphragm and its core-strengthening partnership.

Interestingly, the diaphragm also has a role in controlling intra-abdominal pressure. This pressure regulation is vital for various bodily functions, such as digestion and bowel movements. When you laugh heartily, sneeze, or give birth, your diaphragm helps manage this pressure, ensuring everything stays in its proper place.

Maintaining a healthy diaphragm is essential. Regular deep breathing exercises can help keep this muscle in top shape. By practicing deep, diaphragmatic breathing, you not only enhance your lung capacity but also strengthen your core naturally. It's like giving your parachute a regular check-up to ensure it's always ready to deploy when needed.

In some cases, individuals may experience diaphragmatic hernias, where part of the stomach protrudes through the diaphragm into the chest cavity. While this condition is relatively rare, it can cause discomfort and breathing difficulties. Fortunately, medical interventions, such as surgery, can correct these issues and restore the diaphragm's functionality.

Transverse Abdominis

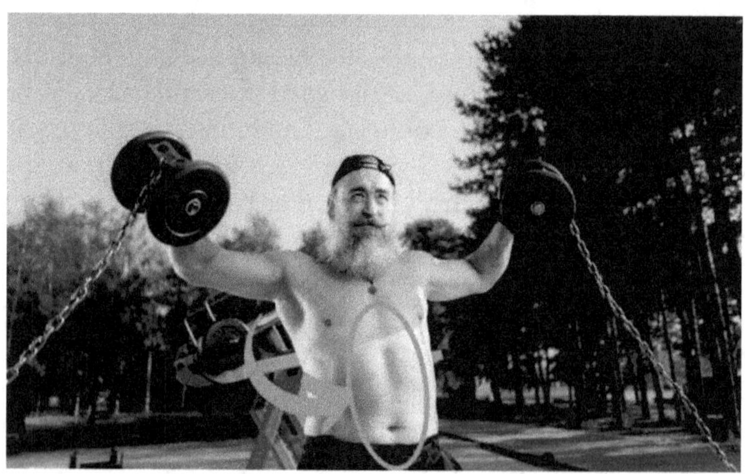

https://www.pexels.com/photo/shirtless-man-lifting-dumbbells-6293101/

The Transverse Abdominis (TVA) is often referred to as your body's built-in weight belt, and it plays a crucial role in supporting your core and safeguarding your spine. This muscle is like a hidden gem within your abdomen, and understanding its significance can greatly benefit your overall health and fitness.

Located deep within your abdominal wall, the TVA wraps around your midsection, similar to how a corset hugs the waist. Its unique positioning allows it to function as a natural girdle, providing stability and support to your spine and pelvis. But that's not all; let's dive deeper into what makes the TVA so remarkable.

One of the primary functions of the TVA is to compress the abdominal contents, which includes your organs, and to keep them in place. This compression not only aids in maintaining good posture but also helps in preventing injury during various physical activities. Whether you're lifting heavy objects, engaging in sports, or simply sitting up straight, the TVA is at work to provide that essential stability.

Now, you might be wondering how to activate and strengthen this hidden powerhouse. Unlike many other muscles, the TVA isn't visible from the outside, making it challenging to target through traditional exercises. However, there are specific techniques that can help you engage and strengthen it effectively.

One such technique is the "drawing-in maneuver." To perform this exercise, imagine pulling your navel toward your spine while maintaining a relaxed breath. It's a subtle movement, and you may not see any visible change, but you will feel a deep contraction in your lower abdomen. Regular practice of this maneuver can help improve the strength and endurance of your TVA.

A strong TVA isn't just about aesthetics; it's also crucial for preventing lower back pain. When this muscle is weak, it can lead to poor posture, which in turn places excessive stress on your lower back. By strengthening your TVA, you can help alleviate and even prevent such discomfort.

Moreover, a well-developed TVA contributes to improved balance and stability. Whether you're an athlete looking to enhance your performance or simply someone who wants to move through daily life with ease, a strong TVA is your secret weapon!

Multifidus

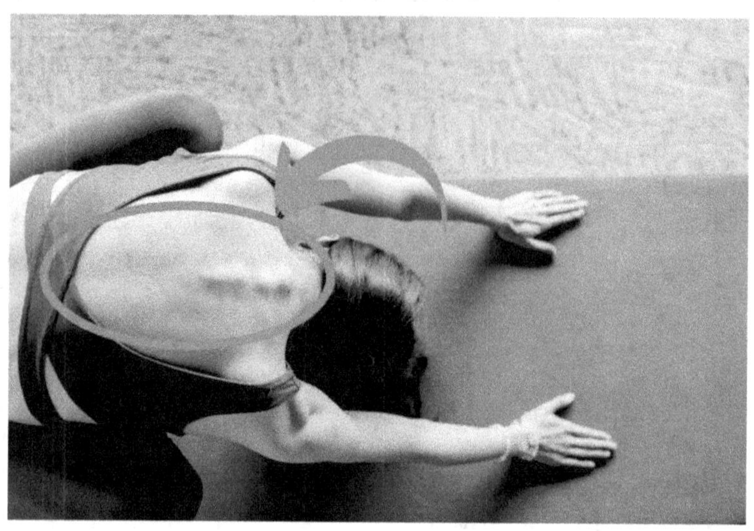

The Multifidus muscles, though small in size, play a colossal role in supporting your spine and facilitating its movement. Picture them as the unsung heroes working tirelessly behind the scenes for your back's well-being. These remarkable muscles are situated alongside your vertebrae, acting as steadfast guardians of spinal stability while also being instrumental in enabling those graceful twists and turns.

When it comes to your spine's well-being, the Multifidus muscles deserve a standing ovation. They are part of a group known as the "deep core" muscles, nestled deep within your back, closer to the spine than the surface. These muscles are not about making you look like a bodybuilder; instead, their mission is to keep your spine strong, steady, and agile.

One fascinating aspect of the Multifidus muscles is their incredible adaptability. They automatically engage when needed, working in tandem with the larger muscle groups around them to provide precise support. When you bend forward to pick up a dropped pen or twist to look over your shoulder while driving, the Multifidus muscles spring into action, helping your spine maintain its proper alignment.

Maintaining strong and healthy Multifidus muscles can be crucial in preventing back pain and injuries. These muscles are like the foundation of a sturdy building, ensuring that your spine stands tall and supports your body's weight effectively. When they are weak or neglected, your spine can become vulnerable, leading to discomfort or even more serious issues.

A lesser-known fact about the Multifidus muscles is that they can also be involved in chronic back pain. When injuries or conditions affect these muscles, it can lead to pain and discomfort that lingers over time. Physical therapists often focus on rehabilitating the Multifidus muscles as part of their treatment plans for individuals dealing with persistent back pain.

Internal and External Obliques

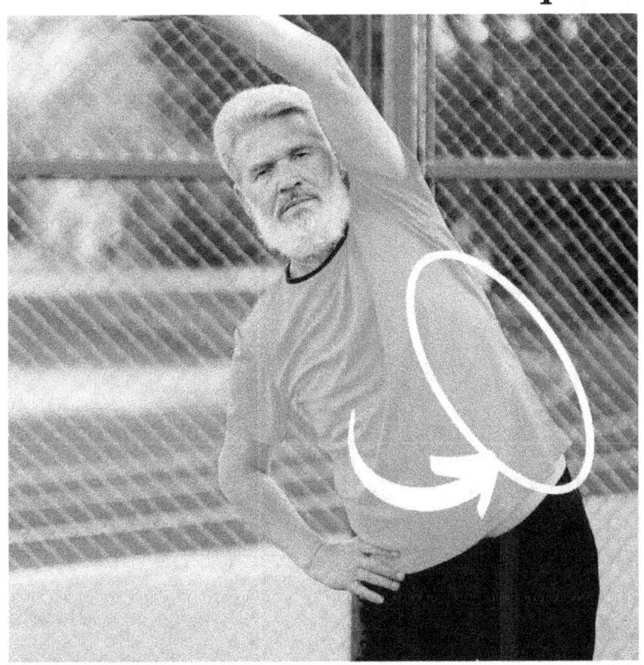

https://www.pexels.com/photo/mature-man-stretching-body-on-sports-ground-5067941/

When it comes to moving your body in a twist-and-turn motion, think of your Internal and External Obliques as the superheroes of your core muscles. They're like the gears in a clock, working together seamlessly to help you reach for that sneaky item lurking behind you. But let's dive deeper into these remarkable muscles and uncover their hidden powers.

Internal Obliques, located deep within your abdomen, are like the body's secret agents. They run diagonally, originating from the lower three ribs and attaching to the iliac crest of the pelvis. These muscles have an essential role in trunk rotation and lateral flexion. When you twist to grab something from the backseat of your car or swing a golf club, these covert muscles spring into action.

Now, let's not forget about their partner-in-crime, the External Obliques. These guys are the surface-level superheroes, easily visible on the sides of your abdomen. They run in the opposite direction of their internal counterparts, originating from the lower ribs and attaching to the linea alba and the pelvis. The External Obliques work hand in hand with the Internals, and they're responsible for actions like bending to the side and rotating your torso.

But wait, there's more! These oblique muscles are not just about twisting and turning; they have other essential functions, too. They provide stability to your spine, protecting it from excessive movement and potential injuries. Imagine them as the body's natural corset, keeping everything in place and supporting your lower back during heavy lifting or when you're doing a tricky yoga pose.

These muscles are also crucial for good posture. Weak obliques can lead to slouching, which can result in back pain and poor alignment. By keeping your Internal and External Obliques in top shape, you're not only enhancing your ability to perform daily tasks with ease but also maintaining a healthy and upright posture.

How do these parts work together?

Understanding how the core muscles work together is like unraveling the secrets of a superhero team, with each member playing a crucial role in maintaining your body's strength and stability. So, let's dive deeper into this fascinating coordination of muscles that makes everyday movements seem effortless.

First, there is the Transversus Abdominis (TVA), the unsung hero of your core. It wraps around your abdomen like a snug belt. When you pick up that heavy box, your brain calls upon the TVA to tighten up. Its job? To provide a solid foundation for your spine, keeping it safe and steady.

Now, let's not forget the diaphragm, your body's built-in breathing coach. When you engage your core, the diaphragm steps in to ensure your breathing remains stable and controlled. It's like having an expert conductor orchestrating your breath, allowing you to focus on the task at hand.

Meanwhile, the multifidus, a series of small but mighty muscles that run along your spine, is quietly doing its part. Its role is to support and stabilize your spine during movements, making sure you maintain proper alignment.

But the core isn't all about these hidden heroes. Your abs and back muscles are the dynamic duo of the core world. They come together in perfect harmony when you lift that heavy box. Your abdominal muscles contract, providing the power needed to lift, while your back muscles work diligently to support your spine and prevent injury. It's like a synchronized dance of strength and balance.

Now, let's talk about the practical side of things. Your core isn't just for lifting boxes; it's your body's central hub for everyday activities. Whether it's sitting up straight at your desk, going for a walk, or even standing in a never-ending line, your core muscles are hard at work.

A strong core is your body's armor against injuries. It acts as a protective shield, reducing the risk of strains and sprains. Additionally, it's your best friend when it comes to maintaining good posture. A robust core effortlessly supports your spine, helping you stand tall and confident.

Chapter 3: Safety First

One critical aspect of overall health is maintaining core strength, which is essential for stability, balance, and functional independence. Core exercises, such as abdominal crunches, planks, and leg raises, are commonly incorporated into fitness routines to strengthen the muscles that support the spine and pelvis.

However, what many may not realize is that the physiological considerations for older adults are significantly different from those of younger individuals. This key distinction underscores the importance of informing older adults about the unique physiological considerations they must take into account before safely performing core exercises.

The aging process brings about a multitude of changes in the body, including alterations in muscle mass, bone density, joint flexibility, and cardiovascular capacity. These age-related changes can have a profound impact on an individual's ability to engage in physical activities, particularly core exercises.

Therefore, older adults must understand how these physiological changes affect their ability to perform core exercises safely and effectively. In this context, a tailored approach to core training that takes into account the specific needs and limitations of elderly individuals is essential for promoting their overall health and quality of life.

In this discussion, we will explore the unique physiological considerations that older adults should be aware of when engaging in core exercises. By doing so, we aim to empower older individuals with the knowledge they need to make informed decisions about their fitness routines, reduce the risk of injury, and maximize the benefits of core strengthening exercises in the context of aging gracefully and healthily.

Bones That Bear Witness to Time

Bones are incredible structures in our bodies, like the strong scaffolding of a skyscraper. When we're young, they're tough and sturdy, just like that skyscraper's frame. But as we get older, our bones go through changes. It's like they're leaving clues about the passage of time in our bodies.

One of the most common changes is a decrease in bone density. You can think of bone density as how tightly packed and strong your bones are. In youth, it's like a solid block of concrete, but as you age, it becomes more like a sponge. This reduction in bone density makes your bones more delicate and prone to breaking.

To comprehend why bones lose density in old age, we must first grasp the fundamental structure of our bones. Think of them as a complex, living framework composed mainly of two key components: minerals and proteins. Calcium and phosphate minerals form the sturdy foundation, akin to the steel in a building, while collagen proteins act as the flexible mortar, providing resilience.

In our youthful years, our bodies are masters at maintaining a delicate balance between building and breaking down bone tissue. This balance ensures that our bones remain robust and can adapt to various stresses and strains. But as we age, this equilibrium can tip in favor of bone breakdown, leading to a decrease in bone density. Why does this happen?

Hormones: One key player in this bone-density drama is our hormones, especially estrogen and testosterone. These hormones have a significant impact on bone health. In women, estrogen levels drop sharply during menopause, leading to accelerated bone loss. For men, a gradual decline in testosterone also contributes to bone density reduction. These hormonal shifts can weaken the bone-building process.

Age: Another culprit in the bone density decline is a natural process called "bone remodeling." Imagine your bones as a bustling construction site. Old bone tissue is continuously being demolished by cells called osteoclasts, while osteoblasts are constructing new bone. In our younger years, the balance leans more toward bone formation. But as we age, this equilibrium tilts, with osteoclasts outpacing osteoblasts, resulting in a net loss of bone density.

Lack of physical activity: Bones, like muscles, thrive when they face resistance and strain. Regular weight-bearing activities (such as walking, jogging, or lifting weights) stimulate the bone-forming cells to do their job. However, inactivity can lead to bone weakening, making them more susceptible to fractures.

Nutrition: is another essential element in the bone density equation. Calcium, vitamin D, and other nutrients are like the construction materials required for building strong bones. A diet lacking in these nutrients can hinder bone health, especially as we age and our bodies become less efficient at absorbing these vital elements.

Medical conditions: Furthermore, certain medications and medical conditions can accelerate bone loss. Long-term use of corticosteroids, for instance, can weaken bones, as can conditions like rheumatoid arthritis, which triggers an inflammatory response that can affect bone density.

Genetics: also plays a role. Some individuals may inherit a higher risk of osteoporosis and reduced bone density from their parents. While we can't control our genetics, understanding this risk can help us take proactive measures to maintain bone health.

When it comes to keeping your core strong, having weak bones doesn't mean you have to sit on the sidelines. With some simple strategies and awareness, you can safely perform core exercises that support your overall health!

Muscle Matters

Muscles, those mighty engines driving our bodies, play a pivotal role in our daily lives. They are the unsung heroes behind every move we make, from getting out of bed to lifting a bag of groceries. When we're young, our muscles are like superheroes, robust and ready for action. They let us carry heavy loads, run, jump, and lead active lives. But, as the years go by, these once-mighty muscles begin to weaken, and it's a natural part of aging.

Now, you might wonder why our muscles weaken as we age. Well, there are a few reasons for this natural decline. One of the primary reasons for muscle weakening with age is the decline in muscle mass. This process, known as sarcopenia, starts as early as your 30s but becomes more noticeable as you get older. It's like your muscles are slowly saying, "I'm taking a break."

Changes in Muscle Fiber: Muscles are made up of tiny muscle fibers. These fibers play a crucial role in muscle contraction and strength. As we age, these muscle fibers become smaller and fewer in number, making it harder for our muscles to generate the force they used to.

Reduced Hormone Production: Hormones like testosterone and growth hormone are essential for muscle growth and maintenance. Unfortunately, as we age, our bodies produce fewer of these hormones. It's like the muscle-building crew is downsizing.

Less Physical Activity: Many people become less active as they age, which can contribute to muscle weakening. When you use your muscles less, they become less robust. So, staying active is like a secret weapon against muscle aging.

Nutrient Absorption: Your muscles need the right nutrients to stay strong. But as you age, your body may not absorb these nutrients as efficiently. It's like your muscle-building materials are getting lost in transit.

Nerve Function: Nerves send signals to your muscles, telling them when to contract. With age, nerve function can decline, leading to reduced muscle activation. It's like a miscommunication between your brain and muscles.

Inflammation and Oxidative Stress: Chronic inflammation and oxidative stress can damage muscle tissue over time. These processes become more common as we age, adding to muscle weakness. It's like your muscles are under constant attack.

Loss of Elasticity: Your muscles are like rubber bands, stretching and contracting as needed. But with age, they lose some of their elasticity, making it harder to generate force. It's like trying to pull a worn-out rubber band.

Medications and Medical Conditions: Certain medications and medical conditions can also contribute to muscle weakness. It's like adding extra weight to your muscles, making them work harder to function.

Lifestyle Choices: Smoking, excessive alcohol consumption, and an unhealthy diet can accelerate muscle aging. These lifestyle choices can damage muscle tissue and hinder its ability to stay strong. It's like throwing obstacles in your muscle's path.

Now, while the natural aging process does bring these muscle changes, it's not all doom and gloom. There's good news! We can take steps to slow down this muscle aging process and even reverse some of the effects. One of the most effective ways to do this is through regular core exercises.

The Dance of Flexibility

Flexibility, the ability to bend, stretch, and twist with ease, is like a graceful dance in our younger years. Our bodies move effortlessly, and reaching for that top shelf is a breeze. However, as the sands of time trickle down, our bodies may lose some of that limberness. Joints start to creak, and even the simplest of movements can become a challenge. It's a natural part of the aging process, but there's more to this story than meets the eye.

Imagine reaching for a jar of your favorite cookies on the top kitchen shelf, and suddenly, you feel a twinge in your back. That's your body sending a signal that it's not as flexible as it used to be. Reduced flexibility is one of the companions of aging, and it can be a bit like a dance partner who starts to step on your toes.

Why does this happen? Well, it's a combination of factors. First up, it's all about collagen. Collagen is like the glue that holds our body together, and it's a vital player in our skin's elasticity. When we're young, our bodies are collagen factories, churning out the good stuff like there's no tomorrow. But as we age, this factory starts to slow down. The result? Skin loses its bounce, and muscles and tendons become less elastic. Think of it as your body's way of saying, "I've been around the block a few times."

Joint Health: Your joints are like the hinges on a door. They allow movement in many directions, but they also wear down over time. As we age, the lubricating fluid in our joints may decrease, making them less smooth and causing friction. This can lead to conditions like arthritis, which can be a flexibility buzzkill. Keep those joints happy by staying hydrated, maintaining a healthy weight, and doing exercises that promote joint mobility.

Inactivity Takes Its Toll: You know that old saying, "Use it or lose it"? Well, it's true. When we lead a sedentary lifestyle, our muscles and joints don't get the regular workout they need. This lack of movement can cause them to stiffen up. So, if you find yourself spending more time on the couch than on your feet, it's time to rethink your habits. Incorporate simple stretches and movements into your daily routine to keep things limber.

Scar Tissue and Adhesions: Remember that time you tripped and scraped your knee? Your body healed it with tough scar tissue. But over time, if you keep getting little injuries or not moving that joint much, that scar tissue can build up and restrict movement. This is how adhesions form, making it harder for your body to move smoothly. Regular stretching can help break up these adhesions and keep you feeling limber.

Nervous System Changes: Our nervous system controls our muscle contractions and movements. As we age, there can be changes in nerve function that affect our flexibility. Nerves may transmit signals more slowly, leading to reduced reaction times and agility. That's why staying mentally and physically active can help keep those nerve pathways firing on all cylinders.

Now, you might wonder, why does flexibility matter? Reduced flexibility isn't just about making reaching for that cookie jar a bit tricky. It can have more serious consequences. One of the biggest concerns is an increased risk of falls and injuries. When your body can't move as it once did, maintaining balance becomes a delicate act.

But having weak bones and muscles – or even reduced flexibility – doesn't mean you can't work on your core strength safely. In fact, it's even more crucial to exercise with caution to avoid injuries. In this guide, we'll explore how to perform core exercises safely when you have weak muscles.

Consulting a Professional

Before embarking on a new core exercise routine, it's crucial to prioritize your well-being by seeking guidance from a healthcare professional or a certified fitness trainer. These experts possess the knowledge and experience needed to assess your unique circumstances and create a fitness plan that aligns with your specific needs and goals.

Why is consulting a professional so important? Let's break it down.

First and foremost, your health matters. By consulting a professional, you ensure that the exercises you undertake won't jeopardize your physical condition. They can evaluate your medical history, identify any underlying health issues, and determine if you have any specific limitations or restrictions that should be considered in your workout plan.

Moreover, these professionals can tailor your core exercise routine to suit your individual requirements. No two bodies are exactly alike, and what works for one person may not be suitable for another. A customized approach takes into account your strengths, weaknesses, and fitness level, ensuring that you're on the right track right from the beginning.

Additionally, a professional can help you set realistic and achievable fitness goals. Whether your aim is to strengthen your core for improved posture, alleviate lower back pain, or enhance your athletic performance, they can create a roadmap that outlines the steps you need to take to reach your objectives safely and effectively.

Safety is paramount when it comes to core exercises. Without proper guidance, you might inadvertently perform exercises with incorrect form, increasing the risk of injury. Professionals not only teach you the right techniques but also monitor your progress to make necessary adjustments as you advance.

Furthermore, they can introduce variety into your routine, preventing boredom and plateaus. Mixing up your exercises keeps your workouts engaging and challenging, ensuring you stay motivated on your fitness journey.

But where can you find these knowledgeable professionals? Start by consulting your primary care physician. They can provide recommendations or referrals to certified fitness trainers or physical therapists who can assist you in your fitness quest. Alternatively, you can explore local gyms, fitness centers, or online platforms that offer access to certified trainers and healthcare experts.

Remember that consulting a professional isn't a one-time affair. It's an ongoing partnership. As your fitness level evolves and your goals shift, they will be there to adapt your core exercise routine accordingly, ensuring you continue to make progress and avoid setbacks.

Start Slow and Gentle

Starting your core exercise routine with a slow and gentle approach is not just a wise choice; it's essential for long-term success. In this guide, we'll explore why beginning with simple exercises, such as pelvic tilts and leg raises, is the key to unlocking your core's full potential.

Core muscles play a pivotal role in stabilizing your body, supporting your spine, and enhancing your overall strength. Jumping headfirst into intense core workouts might seem tempting, but it can lead to injuries and discouragement if you're not adequately prepared.

When you commence your core journey with gentle movements, like pelvic tilts, you're giving your core muscles a chance to wake up without overwhelming them. These movements engage your lower abdominal muscles, helping you establish a strong foundation.

Leg raises are another excellent choice for beginners; these raises target not only your lower abs but also your hip flexors. By including leg raises in your initial routine, you're introducing variety while keeping things manageable. Remember, variety is key to preventing boredom and plateaus in your fitness journey.

But why should you start slow? Here's the deal: Your core muscles may not be accustomed to regular exercise, and they need time to adapt. Rushing into strenuous exercises can lead to soreness, potential injuries, and – worst of all – *demotivation.*

Gradual progression is the secret sauce here. Once you feel comfortable with your chosen gentle exercises, it's time to gradually up the ante. Add more repetitions or extend the duration of your sets. For example, if you were doing ten pelvic tilts, consider aiming for fifteen or twenty as you gain strength.

You can also explore other beginner-friendly core exercises, such as planks or bird-dog. Planks work your entire core and help build endurance, while bird-dog exercises improve balance and stability. These exercises complement your initial routine and provide a well-rounded core workout.

Remember, patience is your ally on this journey. Your core won't transform overnight, but with consistent effort, you'll witness remarkable progress. Track your workouts and celebrate even the smallest victories, such as holding a plank for a few extra seconds or completing an extra set of leg raises.

Proper form is paramount during core exercises. Make sure your movements are controlled and your core muscles are engaged. This not only maximizes the benefits but also reduces the risk of injury.

Incorporating core exercises into your fitness routine offers numerous advantages beyond aesthetics. A strong core can alleviate back pain, improve posture, and boost athletic performance. It's the cornerstone of a healthy and functional body.

Focus on Form

Maintaining proper form is not just a suggestion but a crucial aspect of your core exercise routine. It's the foundation upon which you build strength and stability and avoid potential injuries. So, let's delve deeper into the importance of form and some tips to help you achieve it effortlessly.

First and foremost, let's talk about posture. When you embark on your core exercise journey, posture becomes your guiding star. Imagine a straight line running from your head down to your heels; this is the alignment you want to maintain. Your back should be perfectly straight, and your shoulders should be relaxed. This alignment ensures that your spine is in a neutral position, reducing the risk of strain.

Engaging your core muscles is the next vital step. Your core consists of more than just your abs; it includes your lower back, obliques, and pelvic muscles, too. To engage them effectively, draw your belly button toward your spine. This action activates all the muscles in your core, creating a strong foundation for your exercises.

Now, let's address two common mistakes: arching and rounding your back. Arching your back during exercises like planks or bridges can lead to discomfort and even injury. It places excessive strain on your lower back and can cause pain. On the flip side, rounding your back, especially during exercises like sit-ups, can also result in discomfort and reduced effectiveness of the exercise. It's crucial to keep that spine neutral to protect your back and get the most out of your workout.

As you focus on form, remember to breathe. It might seem obvious, but many people forget to breathe properly during core exercises. Inhale deeply before starting the movement, and as you exert effort, exhale. This controlled breathing not only helps with stability but also ensures you're getting enough oxygen to power through your routine.

Use Supportive Equipment

When embarking on a journey to strengthen your core, one key aspect that often goes unnoticed is the use of supportive equipment. These handy tools, such as exercise mats and stability balls, can be your best companions in achieving a strong and toned core. In this guide, we will delve deeper into the importance of incorporating supportive equipment into your core exercise routine.

First and foremost, let's talk about exercise mats. These seemingly simple mats are your secret weapon in ensuring comfort and safety during core workouts. Picture this: you're on the floor, ready to perform a set of challenging exercises, and suddenly you feel discomfort in your back. This is where an exercise mat comes to the rescue. It provides a cushioning layer between your body and the hard floor, reducing the strain on your spine and allowing you to focus solely on engaging your core muscles.

Moreover, exercise mats offer stability and grip. You won't have to worry about slipping or sliding, which can be a common concern when working out on bare floors. With a stable base, you can perform exercises with confidence, knowing that your mat has got your back, quite literally.

Now, let's shift our attention to stability balls. These inflatable wonders are fantastic for enhancing the effectiveness of your core workouts. The beauty of stability balls lies in their ability to engage multiple muscle groups simultaneously. When you perform exercises like planks or bridges on a stability ball, you're not only targeting your core but also engaging your stabilizer muscles, which play a crucial role in balance and overall strength.

Stability balls also add an element of challenge to your routine. Unlike stable surfaces, these balls are, well, unstable. This instability forces your core muscles to work harder to maintain balance throughout the exercises. It's like giving your core an extra push – making your workouts more efficient and yielding better results.

Furthermore, stability balls provide excellent support for exercises that require lying or sitting positions. They help in maintaining the natural curve of your spine, reducing the risk of strain or injury. So, whether you're doing crunches, Russian twists, or leg raises, a stability ball can be your trusted partner in keeping your spine aligned and your core engaged.

Incorporating supportive equipment like exercise mats and stability balls into your core exercise routine is not just about comfort; it's about maximizing the benefits of your workouts. These tools offer a myriad of advantages, including improved comfort, enhanced stability, increased muscle engagement, and reduced risk of injury.

So, the next time you embark on your core workout journey, don't forget to invite your exercise mat and stability ball along. They may seem like humble accessories, but they have the power to transform your core exercises into a more comfortable, effective, and rewarding experience. With these supportive companions by your side, you'll be well on your way to achieving that strong and toned core you've always desired.

Gradually Increase Intensity

Gradually increasing the intensity of your core exercise routine is a key element in achieving a stronger and more resilient core. This gradual progression is essential for avoiding injury and maximizing the benefits of your workouts. In this article, we will delve deeper into the importance of gradually increasing intensity and provide you with some practical tips on how to do it effectively.

First and foremost, it's crucial to understand that your core muscles, like any other muscle group, need time to adapt and grow. If you push yourself too hard or too fast, you risk straining or injuring these muscles. That's why the mantra "slow and steady wins the race" holds true in the world of core strengthening.

So, how can you effectively increase the intensity of your core exercises over time?

Duration: Start by extending the duration of your core workouts. If you've been holding a plank for 30 seconds, aim to increase it to 45 seconds or even a minute. Gradually adding seconds or minutes to your routine challenges your core muscles without overwhelming them.

Frequency: Another way to intensify your core training is by increasing the frequency of your workouts. Instead of doing core exercises twice a week, try incorporating them into your routine three or four times a week. This allows your muscles to adapt and grow stronger.

Variation: Spice up your core routine with a variety of exercises. Instead of sticking to the same routine, incorporate different movements and angles. For example, if you've been doing traditional crunches, try bicycle crunches or leg raises to engage different parts of your core.

Resistance: Gradually add resistance to your exercises. You can do this by using resistance bands or weights. For instance, when doing Russian twists, hold a weight or a heavy book to increase the challenge for your obliques.

Breathe Properly

Proper breathing is not just an afterthought but a vital component of any successful core exercise routine. Neglecting the importance of breathing can hinder your progress and even lead to injury. So, let's dive deeper into how to breathe properly when engaging in core exercises.

Mindful Breathing: The first step is to be mindful of your breath. Before you begin any core exercise, take a moment to inhale deeply through your nose. This initial inhalation helps prepare your body for the upcoming effort.

Exhalation During Exertion: As you start the movement or engage your core, remember to exhale slowly and steadily through your mouth. This exhalation should be controlled and in sync with the effort you're putting in. It's like a natural bracing mechanism for your core muscles.

Spinal Stability: Proper breathing plays a pivotal role in stabilizing your spine. When you inhale deeply and engage your core while exhaling, you create intra-abdominal pressure. This pressure acts as a natural weight belt, supporting your spine and reducing the risk of injury.

Avoid Breath-Holding: One common mistake during core exercises is breath-holding. Holding your breath can increase blood pressure and tension in your body, making the exercises less effective and potentially risky. So, make a conscious effort to avoid holding your breath.

Rhythmic Breathing: Maintaining a rhythmic breathing pattern is essential. Inhale before the effort, and exhale during the effort. For example, if you're doing a sit-up, inhale as you lower your torso and exhale as you crunch upwards. This rhythm helps you stay in control and maximizes the benefits of the exercise.

Stay Relaxed: While engaging your core muscles and focusing on your breath, remember to keep the rest of your body relaxed. Tension in other muscle groups can reduce the effectiveness of the exercise and lead to discomfort.

Practice Makes Perfect: Like any skill, proper breathing during core exercises takes practice. Don't get discouraged if it feels challenging at first. Over time, it will become second nature, and you'll perform your core exercises more efficiently.

Listen to Your Body

Listening to your body is a fundamental aspect of any successful core exercise routine. It's not just about getting those six-pack abs or a strong core; it's also about ensuring your body stays healthy and injury-free throughout your fitness journey. In this guide, we'll delve deeper into why listening to your body matters and how to do it effectively.

First and foremost, understand that your body communicates with you in various ways during and after a core workout. These signals can be subtle, but they are crucial in maintaining your overall well-being. Here's what you need to keep in mind:

Pain and Discomfort: While it's normal to feel some discomfort during a core workout, especially if you're pushing your limits, it's essential to differentiate between discomfort and actual pain. Discomfort is often a sign that your muscles are working, but pain can indicate that something is wrong. If you experience pain, particularly sharp or persistent pain, stop your exercise immediately. Ignoring pain can lead to serious injuries.

Dizziness or Lightheadedness: Feeling dizzy or lightheaded during a core workout is a sign that you might be overexerting yourself. This can happen if you're not breathing correctly or if you're not giving your body enough time to recover between sets. When you experience dizziness, take a break, sit down, and drink water to rehydrate. If it persists, consult with a healthcare professional.

Shortness of Breath: If you find it difficult to catch your breath during core exercises, it's a sign that you may be pushing too hard. Ensure you're breathing steadily and not holding your breath. Proper breathing not only enhances your performance but also prevents excessive strain on your body.

Fatigue and Muscle Soreness: After a core workout, it's normal to feel fatigue and muscle soreness. These are indications that your muscles have been challenged and are adapting. However, if the soreness lasts for an extended period or is severe, it might be a sign of overtraining. Give your body the rest it needs to recover.

Progress Tracking: Pay attention to how your body responds to your core workouts over time. Are you gradually getting stronger and more flexible, or do you feel like you're hitting a plateau? Listening to your body's responses can help you adjust your routine to achieve better results.

In addition to recognizing these signals, it's crucial to consult with a healthcare professional or fitness expert, especially if you're new to core exercises or have any underlying medical conditions. They can provide guidance on the right exercises for your body and any precautions you should take.

Remember: your body is unique, and what works for someone else might not work for you. It's essential to tailor your core exercise routine to your individual needs and abilities. Don't compare yourself to others, and don't push yourself to the point of injury.

Balance Your Routine

A balanced exercise routine is like the secret sauce to achieving exceptional core strength and overall health. It's not just about doing crunches and sit-ups endlessly; it's about crafting a well-rounded fitness regimen that covers all the bases. So, let's dive deeper into this idea of balance and why it's so crucial for your journey to a stronger, healthier core.

Imagine your core as the epicenter of your body's stability and strength. It's not just about having those sculpted abs you see on magazine covers; it's about having a functional core that supports your daily activities, from lifting groceries to improving your posture. To achieve this, you need to go beyond the typical core workouts.

While core-specific exercises like planks and Russian twists are essential, they're just the tip of the iceberg. Incorporating other forms of exercise is like adding layers to your core strength journey. One of the key players in this game is cardiovascular activities. Think brisk walking, running, swimming, or cycling. These exercises get your heart pumping and improve your endurance, which indirectly benefits your core.

When you engage in cardio, your body burns calories, shedding excess fat that might be hiding your core muscles. As the layers of fat melt away, your core becomes more visible and toned. Plus, cardio workouts engage your core to stabilize your body during movement, helping it grow stronger in the process.

But it doesn't stop there. Strength training for other muscle groups is another essential component of your balanced routine. When you work on muscles like your legs, back, and chest, you create a solid foundation that complements your core. These muscles help you maintain proper form during core exercises, reducing the risk of injury.

Moreover, a well-rounded routine prevents muscle imbalances. Focusing solely on core exercises can lead to the overdevelopment of certain muscles, which can result in poor posture and even pain. By targeting different muscle groups, you ensure that your body remains in harmony.

A balanced approach also keeps your workouts interesting and prevents boredom. Variety is the spice of life, and the same applies to your fitness routine. Mixing it up with different exercises not only keeps you engaged but also challenges your core in new and exciting ways.

So, here's a simple blueprint for a balanced exercise routine:

- Dedicate a few days a week to core-specific exercises, such as planks, crunches, and leg raises

- On other days, get your heart rate up with cardio activities like jogging or dancing.

- Don't forget to sprinkle in some strength training, targeting various muscle groups to maintain balance

Rest and Recover

Rest and recovery are crucial aspects of any effective fitness routine, especially when it comes to core exercises. It's not just about how hard you push yourself during workouts; it's also about how well you allow your body to recuperate. In this article, we'll delve deeper into the importance of rest and recovery for your core muscles, providing you with insights on how to optimize your routine for the best results.

Resting is not a sign of weakness but a smart move for achieving your fitness goals safely. When you engage in core exercises, your muscles undergo stress and strain. These exercises put significant demands on your abdominal, oblique, and lower back muscles. To build strength and endurance in these areas, you need to give them time to repair and grow.

Now, you might wonder, "How long should I rest between core workouts?" The magic number is around 48 hours. This doesn't mean you need to become a recluse for two days; it simply suggests that you should avoid targeting the same core muscles within this timeframe. During these 48 hours, your muscles repair microscopic tears caused by exercise, becoming stronger and more resilient.

While you rest specific core muscle groups, you can still engage in other forms of exercise. Mix things up with cardiovascular activities like jogging, cycling, or swimming. These exercises provide a well-rounded fitness routine and give your core muscles time to heal. Remember, your body is a complex machine that benefits from diversity in its workouts.

Rest and recovery aren't limited to just physical rest. Your diet and hydration play a significant role, too. Ensure you're consuming a balanced diet rich in protein, which aids in muscle repair. Stay hydrated, as water is essential for the overall recovery process.

Sleep is when your body works its magic in repairing and rejuvenating. Aim for 7-9 hours of quality sleep each night to support your core muscles' recovery. Poor sleep can lead to increased cortisol levels, hindering muscle recovery and potentially leading to weight gain.

Incorporating rest and recovery into your core exercise routine is not a sign of weakness but a strategy for success. The 48-hour rule, variety in workouts, attentive listening to your body, proper nutrition, and quality sleep are your allies in building a stronger core while avoiding the pitfalls of overtraining. Remember, achieving your fitness goals is not a sprint but a marathon, and rest is an essential part of that journey!

Chapter 4: The Foundations: Basic Core Movements

Imagine building a house without a solid foundation; it would be unstable and prone to collapse. Similarly, strengthening your core without mastering the basics is like building on shaky ground. To ensure your core workouts are safe and effective, start with the fundamentals.

Diaphragmatic breathing

Proper breathing is the foundation of core strength. It is a simple yet incredibly effective way to engage and strengthen the deep abdominal muscles that make up your core. The diaphragm, a large muscle located beneath your lungs, plays a key role in this process.

Diaphragmatic breathing, also known as deep or belly breathing, is a technique that activates the diaphragm and helps build core strength. Here's how to practice it:

Find a Comfortable Position: Start by taking a seat in a cozy chair, ensuring your feet are firmly planted on the ground while maintaining proper posture with a straight back. You can also lie down on your back if that's more comfortable.

Place Your Hand on Your Abdomen: Gently place one hand on your abdomen, just below your ribcage, and the other on your chest.

Inhale Slowly: Take a slow and deep breath in through your nose. As you breathe in, focus on filling your abdomen with air. Your hand on your chest should remain relatively still, while the hand on your abdomen should rise as your belly expands.

Exhale Completely: Exhale slowly and completely through your mouth or nose, emptying your lungs. As you exhale, imagine your diaphragm gently pushing the air out.

Repeat: Continue this deep breathing pattern for several breaths, aiming for a slow and steady rhythm. Inhale for a count of four, hold for a moment and then exhale for a count of four.

As you practice diaphragmatic breathing, you may notice a subtle tightening sensation in your lower abdomen. This sensation is a sign that you are engaging your deep core muscles. Over time, this simple yet effective breathing technique can help strengthen your core muscles, improve posture, and support your overall balance and stability.

To reap the benefits of diaphragmatic breathing, aim to incorporate it into your daily routine. You can do it while sitting at your desk, watching TV, or before going to bed. The more you practice, the more natural it will become, and the stronger your core will grow.

Pelvic Floor Activation

Before we dive into the exercises, let's get acquainted with your pelvic floor. Sit or lie down comfortably, close your eyes, and take a few deep breaths. Now, imagine the area between your pubic bone and tailbone. These are the muscles we're focusing on. If you're unsure, think about the sensation you get when you stop the flow of urine midstream. Those are your pelvic floor muscles at work!

The Elevator Ride: Imagine your pelvic floor as an elevator with four floors. Inhale as you relax, then exhale and engage your muscles slowly, as if you're stopping at each floor of the elevator. As you ascend, tighten the muscles a little more at each level. Finally, release them gradually on the way back down. Repeat this exercise several times to master control.

The Clock Ticks: Visualize a clock beneath your feet, with 12 at your pubic bone and 6 at your tailbone. Contract your pelvic floor muscles as if drawing the clock's hands toward each other. Hold for a few seconds, then release. This exercise enhances coordination and control.

The Sip and Lift: Picture sipping through a straw while lifting your pelvic floor muscles at the same time. As you exhale, tighten these muscles gently, as if you're sipping through a tiny straw. Release as you inhale. Practice this exercise to refine your control and strength.

Engaging your pelvic floor muscles isn't just about avoiding leaks when you laugh or sneeze. It's about maintaining core stability, preventing back pain, and improving your posture. These exercises can also enhance your intimate life, making it a win-win for both men and women.

Neutral Spine

Now, picture this: your spine is as straight as an arrow, maintaining its natural, gentle curves – this is what we call a "neutral spine." It's your body's default position, one that keeps your spine in its healthiest alignment. Why is it so important, you ask?

A neutral spine position reduces the stress on your vertebrae, preventing back pain and minimizing the risk of injuries. It's like giving your spine a warm, protective hug. When you maintain a neutral spine during your daily activities, you stand taller and walk with confidence. Imagine the elegance and vitality that this brings to your life!

A neutral spine engages your core muscles effectively. It's like activating a hidden power source within you, making your core exercises more potent. Now, let's get practical! Here are some simple steps to help you maintain a neutral spine during exercises and daily activities:

Mindful Awareness: The first step is to become aware of your spine's position. Imagine a string pulling your head toward the ceiling and your hips and shoulders aligning naturally.

Engage Your Core: Activate those core muscles by gently drawing your navel toward your spine. This subtle move adds stability and strength to your neutral spine.

Check Your Posture: Whether you're sitting at your desk, standing in line, or lifting a bag of groceries, remember your neutral spine. Avoid slouching and maintain those curves.

Practice Breathing: Breathing deeply and rhythmically not only relaxes you but also encourages your core to work with your neutral spine. It's like a soothing massage for your inner powerhouse.

Seek Professional Guidance: If you're unsure about your form, consider working with a certified fitness trainer or physical therapist. They can provide personalized guidance to perfect your neutral spine.

Posture Awareness

Posture isn't just about looking good; it's about feeling good and staying healthy. It's time to take the "Posture Challenge." Don't worry; it's not as intense as it sounds. First, stand up straight. Yep, right now. Shoulders back, chest out, and chin up. Feel the difference? That's the power of posture awareness! Now that you're tuned in, here's how to be mindful of your posture throughout the day:

Desk Delight: Whether you're working from home or at the office, make your desk setup your posture ally. Adjust your chair To provide assistance for your lower back, and keep your screen at eye level. Sit back and let those shoulders relax. You've got this!

Gadget Guardian: We love our gadgets, but they can be posture's worst enemy. Hold your phone or tablet at eye level to prevent that pesky "text neck." Your neck and spine will thank you for it.

Walk Tall: When strolling through life, imagine a string pulling you up from the top of your head. This mental trick keeps your spine aligned and your posture in check. Plus, it's an instant confidence booster!

Mirror, Mirror: Use mirrors to your advantage. Catch yourself slouching? Straighten up, and remind yourself that you're on a journey to a stronger core.

Buddy System: Enlist a posture buddy – a friend or family member who can gently remind you to stand tall when you start to slouch. It's like having your very own posture cheerleader.

Stretch it Out: Regular stretching sessions, especially for your chest and hip flexors, can do wonders for your posture. Loosen up those tight muscles and give your core the space it needs to shine.

Mindfulness Magic: Incorporate mindfulness exercises into your daily routine. Breathing exercises and meditation can help you stay present and aware of your body's position.

Time to Dance: Put on some tunes and groove to the beat. Dancing is not only fun but also an excellent way to improve your posture. Channel your inner Fred Astaire or Ginger Rogers!

Importance of Foundations

Mastering these foundational movements is like building a strong core "base camp." Here's why it matters:

Proper technique reduces the risk of injury. By mastering the basics, you ensure that you're not placing any strain on your back or other muscles.

Effective Workouts: When your core is properly engaged, your workouts become more effective. You'll feel the burn where it matters, leading to better results.

Increased Confidence: Knowing that you're performing exercises correctly boosts your confidence. You'll be more likely to stick with your routine and see improvements.

Functional Benefits: These foundations translate into everyday life. You'll find it easier to pick up groceries, play with grandchildren, or even tie your shoes.

Progression: Once you've built a strong foundation, you can confidently progress to more challenging core exercises, further improving your strength and stability.

Before we dive into the core-sculpting fun, let's lay the groundwork with some fundamental exercises. These are the building blocks that will set you on the path to a rock-solid core.

Bridges

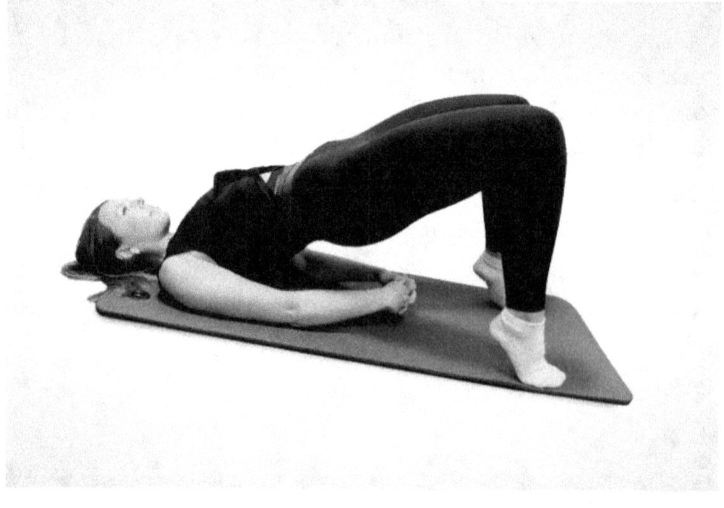

First things first, meet the fundamental move that will be your core's new best friend – the Bridge exercise. Now, don't let the simplicity fool you; this exercise is the real deal when it comes to building a powerful core.

The Setup

First, find a comfortable spot on the floor or a yoga mat. Lie flat on your back with your knees bent and feet flat on the floor, hip-width apart. Your arms should be relaxed at your sides, palms facing down. Make sure your head and neck are in a neutral position, maintaining a small gap between your chin and chest.

The Execution

1. Engage your core muscles, especially those deep abdominals.
2. Take a deep breath in, and as you exhale, press through your heels and lift your hips off the ground.
3. Keep your feet, shoulders, and head grounded as you elevate your hips.
4. Imagine creating a straight line from your shoulders to your knees, forming a bridge-like shape with your body.
5. Hold this bridge position for a few seconds, focusing on the contraction of your glutes and lower back. It's like lifting your core to the sky, inch by inch.
6. You should feel a gentle stretch in your chest and a solid engagement in your core.
7. Keep breathing steadily throughout the exercise.

Key Points

- Engage your core muscles before lifting your hips.
- Maintain a straight line from shoulders to knees.
- Feel the burn in your glutes and lower back.
- Breathe steadily and relax your neck and shoulders.
- Aim for 10-15 seconds in the bridge position as a start, gradually increasing the duration over time.

Common Mistakes to Avoid

- Avoid overextending your back; instead, focus on lifting your hips using your core muscles.

- Don't force your hips too high; aim for a comfortable, controlled lift.

- Remember to breathe! Holding your breath can tense up your muscles unnecessarily.

- Keep your neck relaxed and in line with your spine; don't try to look at your feet.

Now, you might wonder, "Why Bridges?" These exercises are fantastic for seniors because they work not only your core but also your hips, glutes, and lower back – muscles that support your spine and daily movements.

But that's not all! Bridges can enhance your posture, alleviate back pain, and even improve your balance. They're like the Swiss Army knife of core exercises, versatile and effective.

As you embark on your journey to a stronger core, remember that consistency is key. Start with a few reps, gradually increasing as you feel more comfortable. Combine Bridges with other core exercises, and you'll be well on your way to a stronger, more resilient you.

Dead Bug Pose

Let's dive right in with a classic exercise that's both fun and effective: the Dead Bug. Picture yourself lying on your back, ready to embark on a journey to a more resilient core.

The Setup

Before we get into the nitty-gritty, let's set the stage. Find a comfy spot, preferably on a yoga mat or a carpeted floor. Wear loose, comfy clothing that allows for movement, and make sure you have enough space around you.

The Execution

1. Begin by lying flat on your back with your arms extended toward the ceiling. Your knees should be bent at a 90-degree angle, directly above your hips.

2. Tighten your abdominal muscles like you're preparing for a gentle punch to the belly.

3. Keep this engagement throughout the exercise to protect your lower back.

4. Slowly lower your right arm and left leg toward the floor without letting them touch the ground.

5. Keep your core engaged to prevent your lower back from arching off the ground.

6. Bring your right arm and left leg back to the starting position simultaneously.

7. Repeat the movement with your left arm and right leg, lowering them towards the floor without letting them touch.

Key Points

- Breathe naturally throughout the exercise, and don't hold your breath.

- Maintain a steady pace; it's all about control, not speed.

- Feel the tension in your core as you lower your limbs; this is where the magic happens.

- Aim for 10-15 reps on both sides to start, gradually increasing as you get stronger.

Common Mistakes to Avoid

- Keep your lower back glued to the ground throughout the exercise. If it starts to lift, you're losing the core engagement.

- Smooth and controlled is the name of the game. Avoid sudden, jerky motions; it's all about precision.

- Your neck should stay relaxed and in a neutral position. Don't strain it by tucking your chin too close to your chest.

- Always warm up your body before diving into core exercises. A few gentle stretches and mobility exercises will do wonders.

Now that you've got the lowdown on the Dead Bug exercise, it's time to put it into action! This exercise is like a secret weapon for building a stronger core, and as you get the hang of it, you'll feel more stability in your everyday activities.

Seated Tummy Twists

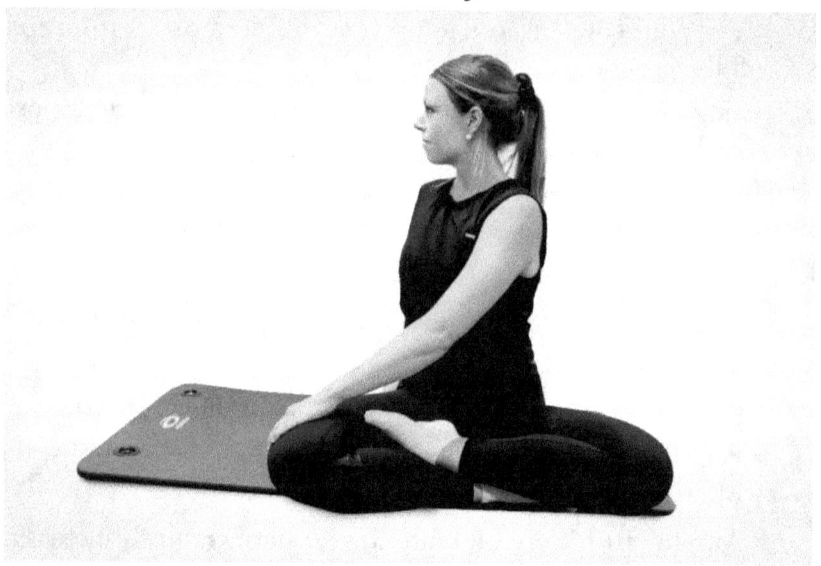

This exercise is like the foundation of a strong core. They're simple, effective, and can be done from the comfort of your favorite chair.

The Setup

Grab a yoga mat and sit up straight, legs crossed. Imagine you're the captain of your ship, ready to take command. Place your hands lightly on your hips, keeping your elbows out. Engage that core like you're bracing for a thrilling adventure.

The Execution

Now, the fun part!

1. Take a deep breath in, and as you exhale, start twisting your upper body to the right. Your head follows your torso's movement.

2. Feel the gentle stretch in your waist. Hold that pose for a moment.

3. Inhale deeply, then exhale as you return to the center.

4. Now, repeat the same to the left side. Picture yourself as a graceful dancer, swaying to a delightful tune.

5. Continue this twisting motion for 10-15 repetitions on each side.

Key Points

- Don't rush; this isn't a race. Savor the movement and engage your core with each twist.
- Remember to breathe in as you return to the center and exhale as you twist. It's the secret sauce that keeps you steady and focused.
- Keep your back straight, and don't slouch. Pretend you're balancing a book on your head.
- Pay attention to the gentle stretch in your waist; that's where the magic happens.

Common Mistakes to Avoid

- Don't push too hard. Start with a few repetitions and gradually increase as your core gets stronger.
- Your chair is your throne; don't hunch over it. Sit tall and proud.
- Remember, inhale at the center and exhale when you twist. It's not just for show; it keeps you balanced.
- Quality over quantity, always. Make each twist count, and don't cheat yourself.
- This is your time to shine. Make it fun, and feel the energy flow.

As you twist away, you're not only building a stronger core but also improving your posture and balance. A strong core means less back pain, better mobility, and a happier you. So, embrace these Seated Tummy Twists, and let your core adventure begin!

Wall Push-Ups

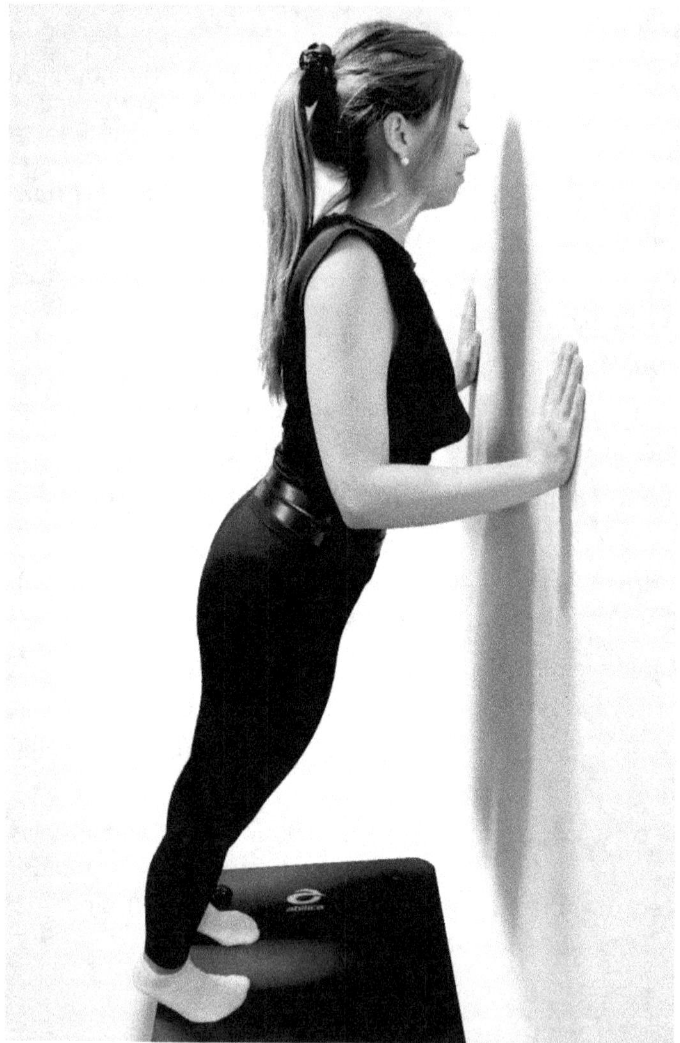

Wall Push-Ups are your secret weapon to a solid core, and they're suitable for everyone, no matter your fitness level. Let's dive into the world of core-strengthening exercises that will leave you feeling invigorated.

The Setup

First, find a sturdy wall, one that won't budge when you lean against it. Stand about arm's length away, feet shoulder-width apart. Plant your feet firmly on the ground; you're rooted like a mighty oak.

The Execution

1. Place your palms flat on the wall, just slightly wider than shoulder-width apart.
2. Your fingers should be pointing upward.
3. Take a deep breath and engage your core muscles.
4. Imagine a string pulling your belly button towards your spine – you're locked and loaded.
5. With a controlled motion, bend your elbows, bringing your chest closer to the wall.
6. Keep your body in a straight line, just like a plank.
7. Don't let your hips sag or stick out – we're aiming for that picture-perfect alignment.
8. Push against the wall to straighten your arms, returning to your starting position.
9. Exhale as you push, feeling the burn in your core. That's the magic happening!

Key Points

- Remember to breathe! Inhale on the way down, exhale as you push up. It helps maintain focus and control.
- Keep your body straight as a board. A strong core depends on maintaining this form. No cheating!
- Start with 8 to 10 repetitions, gradually increasing as you get stronger. Quality over quantity, always.

Common Mistakes to Avoid

- Don't slam your chest into the wall; this is a push-up, not a crash test. Maintain control throughout the movement.
- Keep your neck neutral. Avoid craning your neck forward or letting it hang down; your spine should be in alignment.
- Resist the urge to stick your rear out or let your hips sag. A straight line from head to heel is your goal.

There you have it, the Wall Push-Up – a simple yet powerful exercise that works wonders for your core. Don't let the simplicity fool you; this move engages your core muscles, chest, and shoulders, helping you build a strong foundation for a healthier, more active life.

Plank on Knees

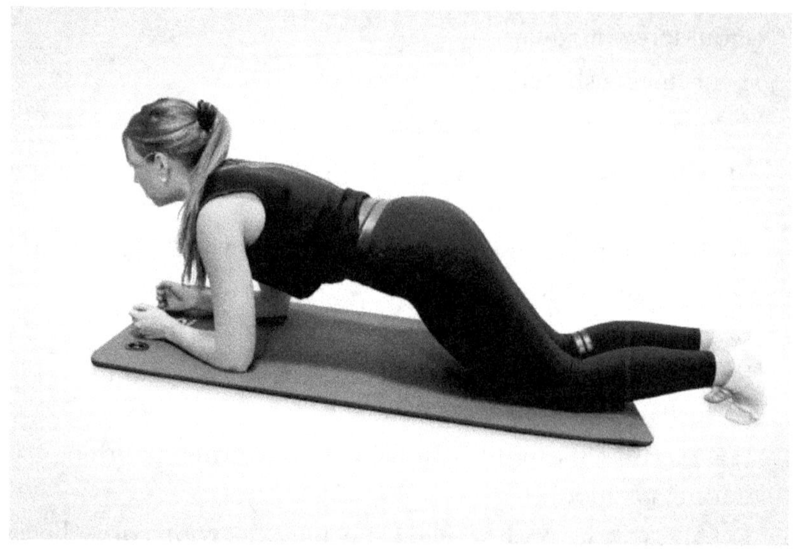

The Plank on Knees is like the gateway to core greatness, specially tailored for beginners like you. Now, I know the idea of planking might make you cringe – *but fear not!* This modified version is here to ease you into it. It's like dipping your toes in the core-strengthening pool before you dive in headfirst.

The Setup

Before we get down to business, let's set the stage. Picture yourself in a cozy, well-lit room, ready to embark on this core-strengthening journey. You don't need fancy equipment or a personal trainer; all you need is a little space and determination.

The Execution

1. Begin by getting down on all fours.

2. Place your hands directly below your shoulders and your knees below your hips.

3. Keep your back flat like a tabletop; this is your canvas for core transformation.

4. Imagine you're pulling your navel towards your spine. This is your secret weapon. Engaging your core stabilizes your spine and lays the foundation for a solid Plank on Knees.

5. Slowly extend one leg back, touching your toes to the ground. Do the same for the other leg.

6. You're now in a modified plank position.

7. Your body should form a straight line from head to knees.

8. Hold this position for 15-30 seconds to start with. As you grow stronger, you can increase the duration.

9. Don't forget to breathe! Inhale deeply through your nose, and exhale through your mouth. Your breath is your ally in this core crusade.

Key Points

- Focus on form, not speed. Slow and steady wins the core race.

- Keep your neck in line with your spine; don't strain it by looking up.

- Contract your glutes and thighs to avoid sagging hips.

- Embrace the shake! Feeling your core muscles working is a sign of progress.

Common Mistakes to Avoid

- If your hips dip towards the floor, it's time for a reboot. Remember to engage those core muscles and maintain a straight line.

- Your back is not a bridge; it should remain flat. Arching can strain your lower back. Keep it in check!

- Don't turn into a breath-holding statue. Breathe rhythmically to keep your body in sync.

- Rome wasn't built in a day, and neither is a stronger core. Avoid overexertion. Start slow and gradually increase your time.

Chapter 5: Why a Strong Core Matters: Posture and Pain

It's a beautiful morning, and you wake up with a stretch and a yawn. You swing your legs out of bed, but as you stand up, a twinge of pain shoots through your lower back. Ouch! It's not the best way to start the day, is it?

Now, imagine this scenario not just for one day but as a daily ritual. Poor posture and nagging pain become unwelcome companions as you navigate your 50s or 60s. But fear not, my friends, because there's a superhero waiting to rescue you – your core!

Let's dive into the fascinating world of core strength, posture, and the relief it can bring.

Poor posture is like a stealthy ninja that sneaks into our lives, causing chaos and discomfort. Think about how we spend hours hunched over our computers, slouched on the couch watching TV, or staring down at our smartphones. It's a posture pandemic!

This constant slumping and slouching puts tremendous strain on our spines. The result? Backaches, neck pain, and even headaches become our daily companions. But there's light at the end of the tunnel – a strong core can be your secret weapon.

But when you build a robust core, it acts as a stabilizer for your spine. Imagine it as a strong support beam, helping you maintain good posture effortlessly. No more slumping! And guess what? Good posture isn't just about looking confident; it's about feeling amazing.

Now, here's where the real magic happens. A strong core isn't just about looking great in a swimsuit (though that's a bonus). It's about being pain-free and full of vitality. As your core strengthens, your spine aligns better, reducing the stress on your back and neck.

Say goodbye to those daily backaches and neck pains. Wave farewell to tension headaches that seem to linger forever. A strong core can be your ticket to a pain-free life in your 50s and 60s.

But how do you get there? What are the secrets to core strength that can transform your life? Well, dear readers, you're in for a treat! In the upcoming chapters, we'll delve into practical exercises, easy routines, and expert advice to help you build a rock-solid core.

So, stay tuned and get ready to embark on a journey towards a pain-free, confident, and healthier you. Your core is your ally, your posture is your armor, and together, they can change your life. Get ready to discover the secrets of why a strong core matters and how it can be the key to unlocking a pain-free, posture-perfect future.

Back Pain – The Silent Saboteur

Back pain is like an uninvited guest that just won't leave the party. It sneaks up on you when you least expect it, making simple tasks like picking up your grandchild or bending to tie your shoelaces feel like Olympic feats. A weak core leaves your spine vulnerable, and when your spine isn't properly supported, it can lead to chronic back pain that feels like an endless battle.

Now, imagine this scenario: you're trying to catch up on your favorite novel, but every few minutes, you have to stop because your neck feels like it's carrying the weight of the world. Neck strain is a common companion of a weak core. Without a strong foundation, your neck muscles work overtime to compensate, leading to those nagging aches and stiffness.

Now, you might be thinking, "Why is this happening to me?" Well, my friends, the culprit here could very well be your weak core muscles. You see, your core isn't just about having killer abs; it's about having the strength to support your entire body, especially your spine.

Let's get real for a moment. Back pain is no joke, and it affects millions of us as we age. But here's the silver lining – strengthening your core can be your secret weapon against it. Don't just take my word for it; let's hear from some folks who've been through it:

Meet Susan, a vibrant 58-year-old who used to suffer from chronic back pain. She said, "I felt like I was trapped in my own body, unable to enjoy life to the fullest. Then, I discovered the magic of core exercises. It was like a game-changer. Not only did my pain subside, but I also felt stronger and more confident."

And then there's Mark, a sprightly 65-year-old who used to grimace with each step he took. He shared his story, saying, "I thought back pain was just a part of getting older. But when I started working on my core, I realized I had the power to turn things around. Now, I walk tall, pain-free, and with a smile on my face."

So, why does a weak core lead to back pain? It's simple. Your core muscles provide essential support to your spine and help maintain proper posture. When they're weak, your spine doesn't get the support it needs, leading to poor alignment and discomfort.

Imagine your core as the strong, dependable friend who's got your back – quite literally! When your core is strong, it acts as a stabilizing force for your spine, preventing excessive strain on your lower back. It's like having your own personal bodyguard against pain.

But don't worry, you don't have to become a gym rat or start doing crazy acrobatics. Simple exercises that target your core muscles can make a world of difference. We'll delve into these exercises and more in the upcoming chapters, so stay tuned!

In a nutshell, your core strength is your ticket to a pain-free, active, and enjoyable life in your golden years. The journey to a strong core and a pain-free back is an adventure worth taking. So, if you're tired of being on the sidelines, it's time to step into the spotlight of a stronger, healthier you.

Neck Strain – The Unwanted Hitchhiker

Let's not forget about the pesky headaches that can ruin a perfectly good day. A weak core can throw your posture off balance, causing tension in your neck and shoulders. The result? Those throbbing headaches that just won't quit. Who wants that kind of party pooper?

Imagine a tent without sturdy ropes holding it up - it starts sagging. Similarly, when your core can't support your upper body, your shoulders and neck bear the brunt of the load. Over time, this can lead to poor posture, and your neck muscles have to work extra hard to keep your head up. Ouch!

But wait, we don't want to scare you with the gloomy side of things. Instead, let's dive into some real-life stories that might hit close to home.

Strengthening your core isn't as daunting as it sounds. Simple exercises like planks, bridges, and seated leg raises can work wonders. It's like giving your core muscles a pep talk, encouraging them to support your neck and shoulders better.

As you embark on this journey to a stronger core, you'll not only bid farewell to neck strain but also welcome better posture, improved balance, and reduced back pain into your life. Who wouldn't want that?

Headaches - The Hidden Havoc of a Weak Core

Headaches, like unwanted guests, come uninvited. They crash your daily routines, dimming your zest for life. But did you know that a weak core might be the culprit behind these unrelenting headaches? Let's dive into this hidden havoc.

Imagine sitting at your desk, staring at the screen, your back hunched, shoulders slouched. You've been in this position for hours, and suddenly, there it is - the headache. It's as if your brain is pounding against your skull, screaming for attention. Sound familiar?

Now, you might be wondering, what does my core have to do with these head-thumpers? Well, picture your core as the sturdy foundation of a skyscraper. If it's weak, the entire structure wobbles, causing stress to ripple through your body.

When your core muscles lack strength, they can't support your spine properly. This leads to poor posture, and poor posture can be a one-way ticket to Headache Land. Your neck and shoulder muscles overcompensate, straining themselves like overworked superheroes. This, my friends, is the beginning of a long-lasting headache saga.

Meet Sarah: "I used to get these excruciating tension headaches every week. It was like a vice grip around my head. Then I started core-strengthening exercises, and voila! The headaches became history."

John's Story: "I thought my headaches were just part of aging. But after some core workouts, they vanished like a magician's trick. Now, I feel better at 60 than I did at 40!"

These real-life success stories are just a glimpse of what's possible when you make your core a priority. So, dear reader, if you're tired of being held back by back pain, neck strain, and those pesky headaches, it's time to take action. Strengthening your core can transform your life, and in the chapters that follow, we'll explore the hows and whys of core strength, providing you with actionable tips and exercises that will leave you standing tall and pain-free in your 50s and 60s.

In the pages that follow, we'll dive deeper into core-strengthening exercises and lifestyle adjustments tailor-made for the seasoned adventurer in you.

Chapter 6: Balance and Stability Exercises for Fall Prevention

Falls among the elderly are far more than mere accidents. They're silent adversaries, lurking in the shadows, waiting for the right moment to strike. Let's explore some compelling statistics and facts that highlight the dangers and consequences of falls in the elderly population, painting a vivid picture of why it's crucial to take action.

A Startling Fact: The Prevalence of Falls

Did you know that falls are the leading cause of both fatal and non-fatal injuries among people aged 65 and older? Each year, millions of older adults experience falls, often resulting in devastating consequences. What's more alarming is that these falls can happen to anyone, anywhere, and at any time.

The Domino Effect: One Fall Leads to Another

Once an elderly individual takes a tumble, it often triggers a chain reaction of fear and immobility. A person who has fallen before becomes more fearful of falling again, which can lead to a significant reduction in physical activity. This sedentary lifestyle can exacerbate muscle weakness and decrease bone density, making future falls even more likely.

The Costly Toll: Economic and Emotional Burden

Falls impose not only a physical burden but also a heavy financial one. Medical expenses, including hospitalization, rehabilitation, and long-term care, add up rapidly. These costs can be especially burdensome for those on fixed incomes. Beyond the financial toll, falls can shatter an individual's self-confidence and independence, causing emotional distress that can linger for years.

Hidden Health Consequences: Fractures and Trauma

When an older adult falls, they are at an increased risk of sustaining fractures, particularly hip fractures. These fractures often require surgery and extended rehabilitation, and sadly, many individuals never fully recover their pre-fall level of function. Moreover, falls can lead to a downward spiral in overall health, increasing the risk of other medical conditions and complications.

A Deadly Threat: Mortality Rates

Falls can have dire consequences, sometimes leading to fatalities. The risk of mortality significantly increases after a fall, particularly among older adults. It's not just the physical impact of the fall itself but also the subsequent health complications that can prove fatal.

Now that we've shed light on the stark realities of falls among the elderly, it's clear that we must take proactive steps to prevent these life-altering incidents. This book is your roadmap to achieving balance, stability, and a strong core – the keys to staying on your feet and enjoying the vibrant life you deserve.

The Core Solution

Without a strong core, the shock of a misstep can jolt through your body like a lightning bolt, causing pain and potential injury. Ouch, right?

But here's where your core comes to the rescue again. It acts as a shock absorber, dispersing the impact of those sudden movements, saving your joints, and keeping you on your feet. When your core is weak, your body has to rely on other muscles to compensate, which can lead to imbalances and increase your risk of injuries. So, if you want to stay active and pain-free, it's time to give those core muscles some love.

Now, let's talk about aging gracefully. We all want to maintain our independence and vitality as we get older, right? Well, a strong core is your secret weapon for achieving just that.

Think of your core as the foundation of your body. When it's solid, you can engage in all the activities you love, from gardening to dancing, without worrying about back pain or stiffness slowing you down. It's like having the key to unlock the door to a more vibrant, pain-free life.

Consistency is your best friend on this journey to a stronger core. Picture it like this: you wouldn't expect to run a marathon after a day of training, right? Similarly, building core strength takes time and commitment. It's not about quick fixes; it's about long-term gains. So, embrace the process, stick to your routine, and watch your core transform.

Now, let's address something we all love to avoid - gradual progression. I get it; we're all eager to see results *yesterday...* but *slow and steady wins the core race.* Think of your core as a delicate flower; you wouldn't want to force it to bloom. Gradual progression not only reduces the risk of injury but also ensures sustainable results. Start with simple exercises and gradually intensify them. Your core will thank you!

Seated Leg Lifts

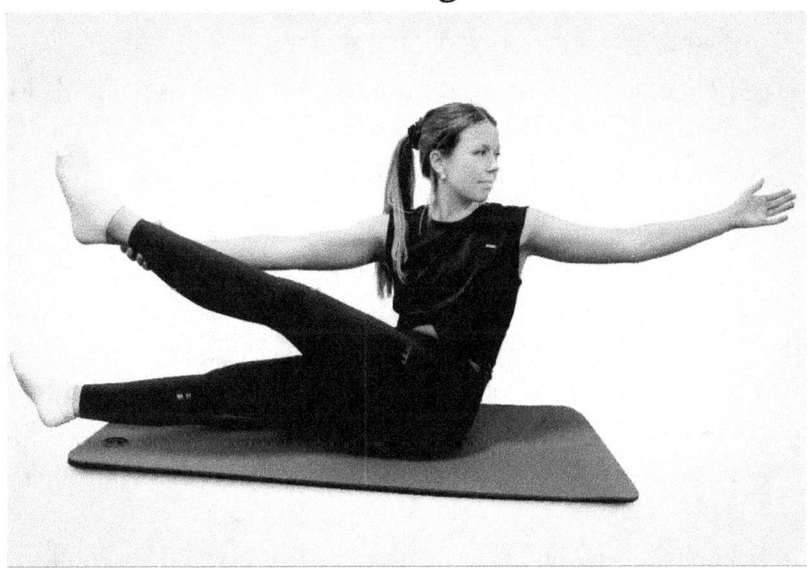

Seated Leg Lifts are like the secret sauce for your core. They target your abdominal muscles, lower back, and hips all at once! When you strengthen these muscles, you're not just improving your posture but also reducing the risk of back pain.

The Setup

Sit on a mat with your legs extended. Take a deep breath in and exhale, engaging your core muscles. This is your starting position – strong and centered.

The Execution

1. Now, lift your right leg straight out in front of you.

2. Keep your toes pointed forward and your knee as straight as possible.

3. Hold it for a few seconds, feeling the burn in your core. Then, slowly lower your leg back down to the ground.

4. Repeat the same process with your left leg.

5. Lift it up, hold it, and lower it down. Imagine your core working like a coiled spring, powering your leg lifts.

6. Remember to breathe steadily throughout the exercise.

7. Inhale as you lift your leg, and exhale as you lower it down. This helps maintain your core stability.

Key Points to Keep in Mind

- Focus on quality, not quantity. Start with a few reps and gradually increase as you build strength.

- Keep your core engaged throughout the exercise. This is where the magic happens!

- Don't rush. Slow and controlled movements are the key to effective Seated Leg Lifts.

- Maintain good posture. Keep your back straight and avoid slouching.

Common Mistakes to Avoid

- It's easy to swing your leg up and down quickly, but this won't engage your core effectively. Control is key.

- Resist the urge to lean your upper body toward your lifted leg. This takes the focus away from your core.

- Forgetting to breathe can lead to tension and discomfort. So remember, inhale and exhale with purpose.

Seated Leg Lifts are your ticket to a stronger core. They might look unassuming, but they are the building blocks to a better, more active life. As you continue practicing this exercise, you'll feel your core becoming more robust, your balance improving, and your overall strength skyrocketing.

Heel-to-toe walks

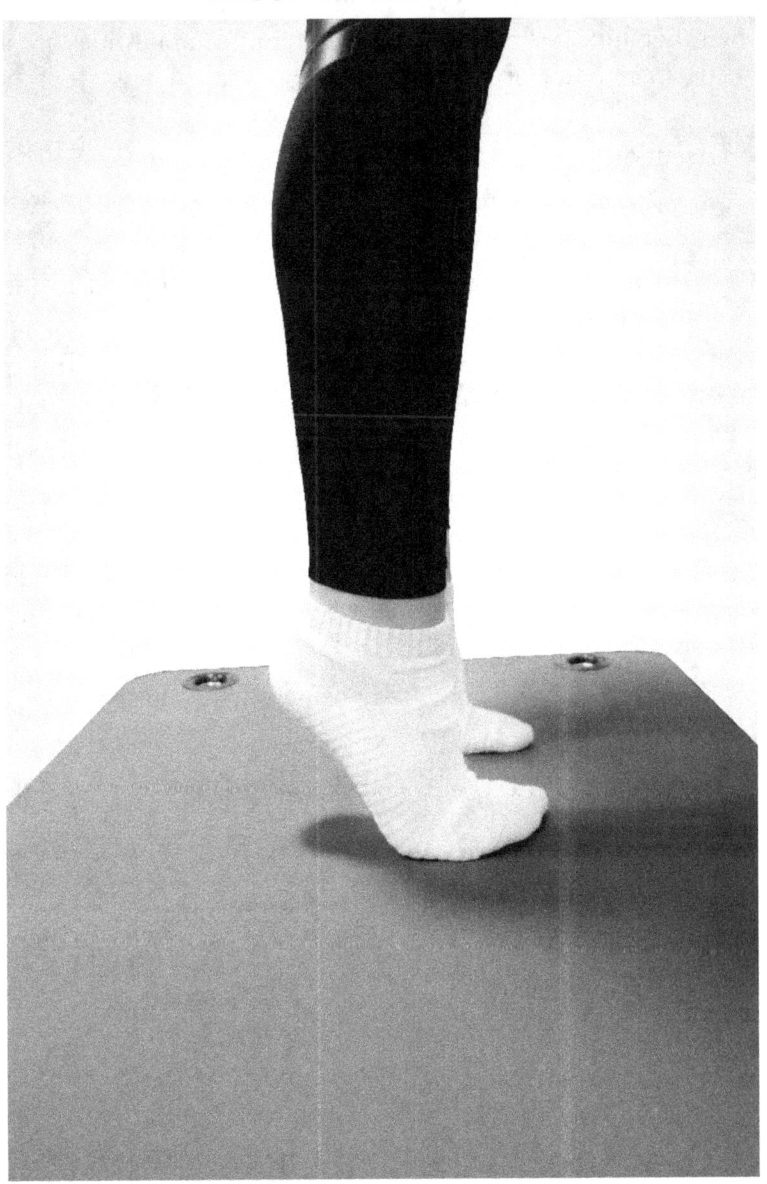

It may seem simple, but this exercise is a core powerhouse. It strengthens not just your core but also improves your balance and stability. As you walk this narrow path, your abdominal muscles engage, supporting your spine and improving posture. Plus, it's a fun way to challenge yourself, and who doesn't love a little challenge, right?

The Setup

To perform Heel to Toe Walks, you won't need fancy equipment or a gym membership. Just a bit of space and comfortable shoes are all you need. Start in a quiet area where you can walk a few steps without obstacles. Begin by standing up straight with your feet together.

The Execution

1. Lift your right heel and place it in front of your left toes. Ensure your feet are in a straight line.

2. Gradually transfer your weight from the right heel to the right toes, pushing off the left toes.

3. Move your left foot forward, placing the left heel in front of the right toes. Keep the line straight and roll through your foot.

4. Continue this heel-to-toe pattern, moving forward with each step. Aim to take at least 10 to 15 steps.

Key Points

- Throughout the exercise, consciously tighten your abdominal muscles. This will help stabilize your body and strengthen your core.

- Focus on keeping your body centered as you shift your weight from heel to toe. Use your arms for balance if needed.

- There's no rush! Walk at a speed that allows you to maintain proper form and balance.

Common Mistakes to Avoid

- Keep your gaze straight ahead to maintain balance. Avoid looking at your feet, as it can throw off your alignment.

- Take your time with each step. Fast, hurried movements can compromise your balance and core engagement.

- Don't slouch or lean forward. Stand tall and proud throughout the exercise.

Standing Leg Lifts

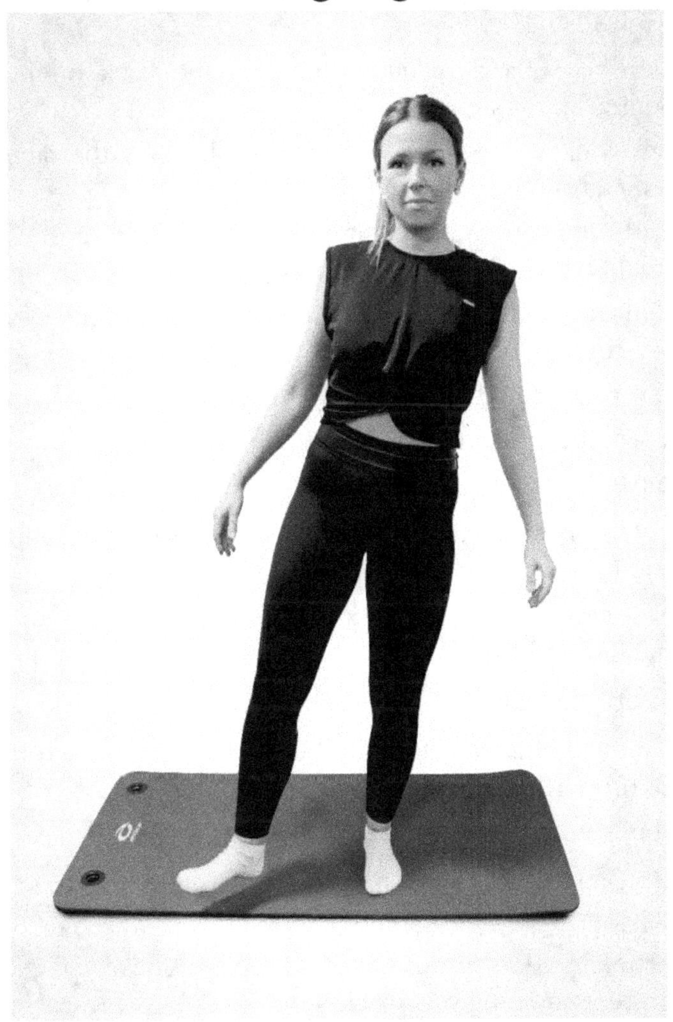

Now, let's dive into one of the foundational exercises - the Standing Leg Lifts. Don't be fooled by its simplicity; this exercise is your ticket to a robust core. It targets those deep abdominal muscles, helping you stand tall and confidently.

The Setup

You don't need fancy equipment or a gym membership for this one. Find a clear space to stand, preferably in front of a sturdy chair or countertop that you can hold onto for balance if needed. Stand up straight, engage your core, and maintain good posture throughout.

The Execution

1. Begin by standing with your feet hip-width apart, toes pointing forward.
2. Keep your hands gently resting on the back of the chair or countertop for support.
3. Shift your weight onto one leg while keeping the other foot flat on the ground.
4. Slowly lift your non-weight-bearing leg off the ground. Keep it straight but not locked at the knee.
5. Hold the lifted leg for a few seconds, feeling the engagement in your core and the stability in your standing leg.
6. Lower your lifted leg back down to the ground.
7. Repeat the exercise on the other side.

Key Points

- Focus on your breath – inhale as you lift your leg and exhale as you lower it.
- Engage your core muscles throughout the exercise to maintain stability and balance.
- Keep your standing knee slightly bent to avoid locking it.
- Gradually increase the number of repetitions as you get more comfortable with the exercise.

Common Mistakes to Avoid

- Don't push yourself too hard. Start with a few repetitions and gradually increase them over time.
- Maintain good posture to get the most out of the exercise and prevent strain on your back.
- Lift your leg in a controlled manner, avoiding jerky movements or swinging.
- Always warm up your body before diving into any exercise routine to prevent injury.

Standing Leg Lifts are fantastic for building core strength, improving balance, and enhancing your overall stability. Remember, Rome wasn't built in a day, and neither is a strong core. Consistency is key, so make it a part of your daily routine.

Pelvic Tilts

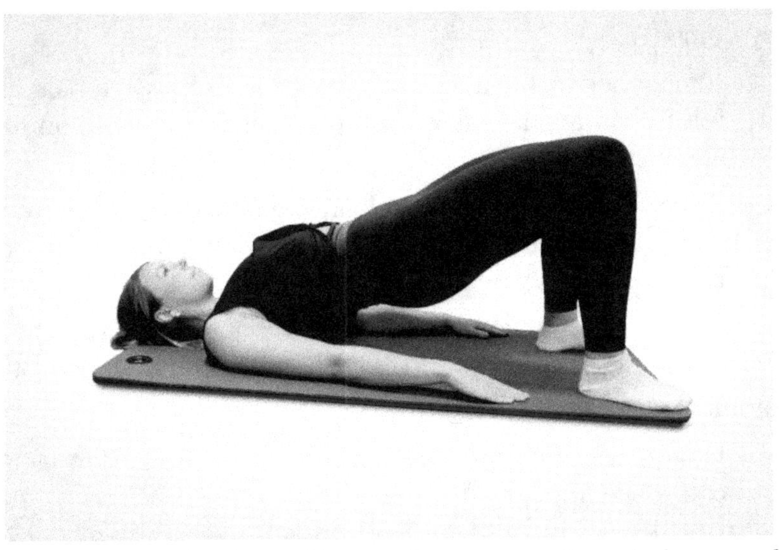

Pelvic Tilts are like the architects of your core. They help you achieve better posture, improve balance, and alleviate lower back pain. Think of them as the invisible superhero cape you wear every day to stand tall and conquer life's challenges.

The Setup

Before we get into the nitty-gritty of Pelvic Tilts, find a comfortable spot. It could be your living room, your backyard, or even your favorite park bench. Wear loose, comfy clothes, and make sure you have a soft mat or towel handy.

Now, lie on your back with your knees bent, feet flat on the ground, and arms resting gently at your sides. Imagine you're preparing for a relaxing afternoon nap. That's the setup – simple, right?

The Execution

1. Take a deep breath in, letting your belly rise, and exhale slowly.

2. As you exhale, press your lower back gently into the floor, tilting your pelvis upward. Imagine tucking your tailbone between your legs.

3. Hold this position for a few seconds, feeling the tension in your core.

4. Then, inhale and release your pelvis back to the starting position.

5. Repeat this movement, focusing on the tilt of your pelvis.

6. You're doing it! Keep it smooth and controlled, like a gentle dance.

Key Points

- Remember to breathe throughout the exercise. Inhale as you release, and exhale as you tilt your pelvis. It keeps you relaxed and engaged.

- Keep the movements slow and deliberate. Rushing won't get you those results you're after. Your core will thank you for your patience.

- Pay attention to your lower back and abdominal muscles. You should sense them working together. That's the sweet spot!

Common Mistakes to Avoid

- Don't exaggerate the arch in your lower back. The goal is a controlled tilt, not a dramatic stretch.

- Breathing is your ally. Don't hold your breath during the exercise. It's your secret weapon for core engagement.

So, why are Pelvic Tilts essential for a stronger core? They lay the foundation by activating your deep abdominal muscles and gently waking up those neglected core muscles. Plus, they improve your posture and provide relief from lower back pain.

Chapter 7: Gentle Flexibility and Mobility Stretches

Flexibility and mobility are like the superheroes of senior health. They swoop in to save the day, making life easier and more enjoyable. So, what's in it for our senior pals when they embrace these superpowers?

Enhanced Daily Functionality: Picture this – effortlessly reaching for that jar of pickles on the top shelf, bending down to tie your shoelaces without a struggle, or simply getting out of bed with a spring in your step. That's the magic of improved flexibility and mobility right there! Seniors who regularly engage in core exercises find it easier to perform everyday tasks, maintaining their independence and zest for life.

Injury Prevention: Let's face it: no one wants to be sidelined by an injury. With age, the risk of slips, trips, and falls increases – but don't worry; having a flexible and mobile body acts as a protective shield. It's like wearing invisible armor. Strong cores and limber muscles stabilize your body, reducing the chances of accidents and injuries.

Pain Relief: Aches and pains are uninvited guests that often show up as we get older. But guess what? Improved flexibility can be your secret weapon against these pesky intruders. By keeping your muscles and joints flexible, you can ease or even prevent discomfort. Say goodbye to those nagging backaches!

Better Posture: Remember when your mom told you to stand up straight? She was onto something! Good posture not only makes you look taller and more confident, but it also helps you breathe better and reduces strain on your back. Flexibility and mobility exercises can help you achieve that elegant posture you've always admired.

Mood Boost: Let's not forget about the mental aspect of it all. When your body feels good, your mind follows suit. Engaging in core exercises that enhance flexibility and mobility can boost your mood, reduce stress, and increase your overall sense of well-being. It's like a happiness cocktail for your body and soul.

Age Gracefully: Embracing flexibility and mobility isn't about defying your age; it's about aging gracefully. It's about living your best life, regardless of the number on your birthday cake. These exercises can help you maintain your youthful spirit and keep you active for years to come.

The Gentle Approach: Safety First

Now, we're all about keeping things easy-breezy here. Our exercises prioritize gentleness above all else. We understand that you might not be training for a marathon, but you still want to enjoy life to the fullest. These routines are tailored to improve your range of motion, reduce stiffness, and do it all without breaking a sweat.

Before we dive into the exercises, remember that safety is non-negotiable. Always consult your healthcare provider before starting any new exercise regimen. They can give you the green light and even offer some personalized tips. Let's kick things off with some delightful stretches to get those joints moving smoothly. The key here is *gentle*. We're going for a luxurious stretch, not a contortionist act!

Cat-Cow Stretch

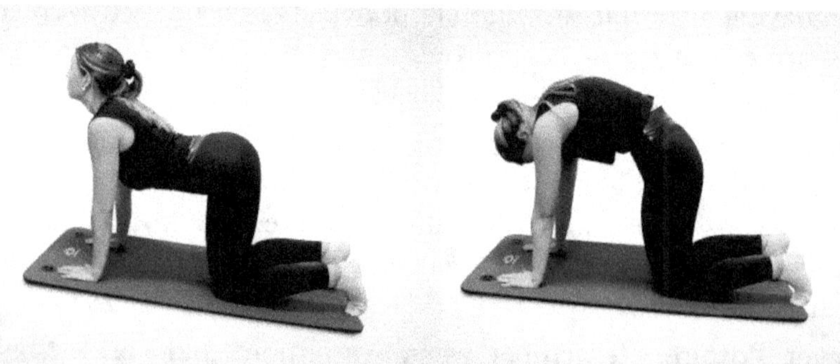

The Cat-Cow Stretch is like a warm hug for your spine. It helps improve flexibility and mobility in your back while also engaging your core muscles. This exercise is perfect for seniors as it's gentle on the joints and can ease those nagging back pains that seem to come out of nowhere.

The Setup

Find a comfortable spot on the floor or a yoga mat. Lower yourself to the ground, positioning your wrists directly beneath your shoulders and your knees beneath your hips.

The Execution

1. Inhale deeply, arch your back up like an angry cat, tucking your chin towards your chest.
2. Imagine you're pulling your belly button toward your spine.
3. Breathe out gradually as you gently curve your back downwards, raising both your head and tailbone toward the sky. Allow your abdomen to descend towards the ground.
4. Repeat this gentle motion, inhaling as you become the "Cat" and exhaling as you transform into the "Cow." Move smoothly and continuously, syncing your breath with your movements.
5. Aim for 10-15 repetitions.

Key Points

- Keep your movements slow and controlled, focusing on the stretch and the breath.
- Engage your core muscles throughout the exercise, maintaining stability.
- Visualize the flexion and extension of your spine with each transition.
- Listen to your body, and don't push yourself into any uncomfortable positions.

Common Mistakes to Avoid

- Don't rush through the Cat-Cow Stretch. It's not a race; it's a mindful exercise.
- Avoid over-arching your back in the Cow position. Keep it gentle and natural.
- Your breath is your guide. Don't forget to sync it with your movements for the full benefits.

Seated Forward Bend

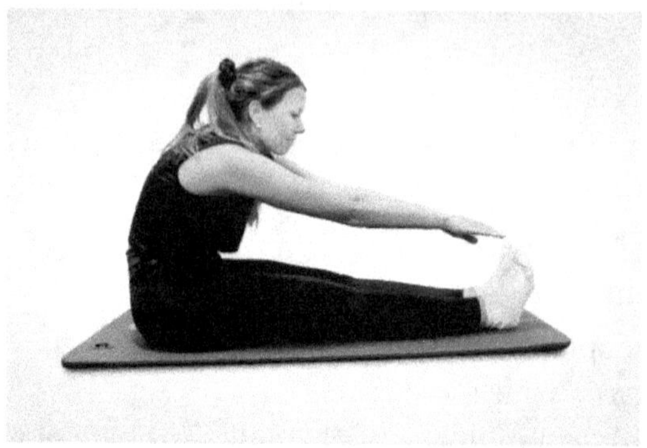

The Seated Forward Bend is your ticket to a more robust core and a healthier you. This exercise is like the foundation of a strong building, setting the stage for a rock-solid core. Let's dive right in and discover how to master it.

The Setup

Sit on a yoga mat with your legs stretched and your feet hip-width apart. Keep your spine tall, and your shoulders relaxed. Reach for your legs, palms facing down.

The Execution

1. Inhale deeply and lengthen your spine as you sit up straight.

2. As you exhale, slowly begin to hinge at your hips, leaning forward from your waist.

3. Keep your back straight and your chest open as you lower your torso towards your thighs.

4. Continue to reach forward until you feel a gentle stretch in your lower back and hamstrings. Don't push yourself too hard.

5. Hold this position for 15-30 seconds, breathing deeply and relaxing into the stretch.

6. To return to the starting position, inhale and engage your core muscles.

7. Slowly roll back up to a sitting position, one vertebra at a time.

Key Points

- Focus on maintaining good posture throughout the exercise. Imagine a string pulling the crown of your head towards the air.

- Breathe deeply and evenly to enhance the stretch and relaxation.

- Feel the stretch in your lower back and hamstrings, but don't force it. Flexibility will improve with practice.

- Keep your abdominal muscles engaged as you lean forward; this activates your core.

Common Mistakes to Avoid

- Avoid hunching or rounding your back during the forward bend. This can strain your spine. Keep your back straight and chest open.

- Don't push yourself too hard in the beginning. Overstretching can lead to injury. Aim for a comfortable stretch that you can hold without pain.

- Remember to breathe! Holding your breath can increase tension in your body, defeating the purpose of the exercise.

- Don't use momentum to go deeper into the stretch. The goal is to engage your core and stretch your hamstrings gradually.

The Seated Forward Bend is like the first step on a stairway to a stronger core. Practice this exercise regularly, and you'll be amazed at how it lays the foundation for a more toned midsection. As you journey deeper into the world of core exercises, you'll discover new challenges and exciting variations to further strengthen your core muscles.

Neck Tilts and Turns

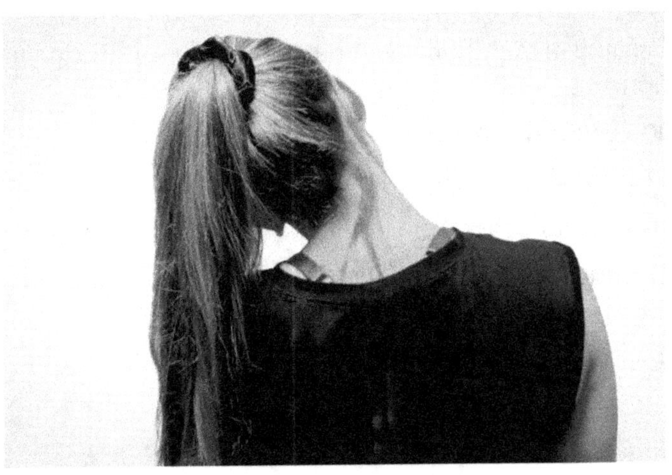

Neck Tilts and Turns may seem simple, but they're the foundational bricks of core strength. By gently tilting and turning your neck, you activate deep core muscles. These exercises improve stability, making everyday activities easier.

The Setup

Before we start, find a comfy chair or stand up straight, feet shoulder-width apart. Relax your shoulders, keep your chin parallel to the floor, and smile – because this is going to be fun!

The Execution

1. Start by inhaling deeply, and as you breathe out, softly incline your head to the right, drawing your right ear nearer to your right shoulder.

2. Maintain the stretch for a brief moment, sensing the tension along the left side of your neck.

3. Slowly return your head to the center.

4. Repeat the tilt, this time to the left side, bringing your left ear closer to your left shoulder.

5. Hold for a few seconds again.

6. Return your head to the center.

7. Repeat this soothing motion 5-10 times on each side.

Key Points

- Keep your movements slow and controlled. Imagine you're moving through warm, thick honey.

- Never force your head down; let gravity do the work.

- Breathe naturally throughout the exercise, and maintain good posture.

Common Mistakes to Avoid

- Don't rush through it like you're in a race. Savor the stretch.

- Avoid hunching your shoulders; keep them relaxed and down.

- Don't tilt your head too far; listen to your body and stay within a comfortable range.

Quadriceps Stretch

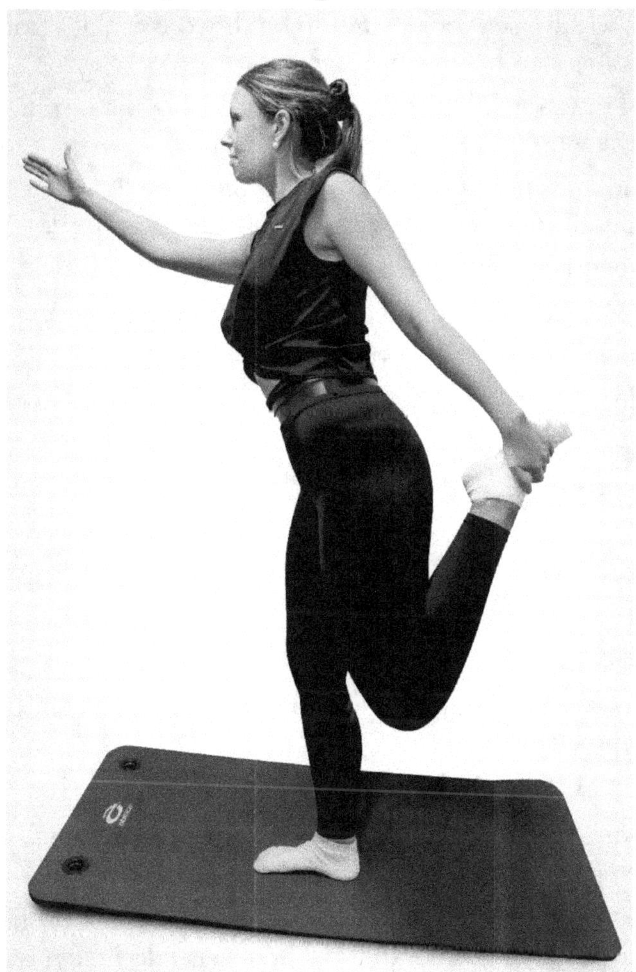

The Quadriceps Stretch isn't just about saying goodbye to tight thighs; it's about strengthening your core's building blocks. By working your quadriceps, you're setting the stage for a more robust and balanced core, which will improve your overall stability and posture.

The Setup

Find a quiet and comfortable spot, preferably with a soft surface like a yoga mat or carpet.

Stand tall with your feet hip-width apart. Ensure you're in a balanced and relaxed position before we dive into this energizing stretch.

The Execution

1. Begin by gently lifting your right foot off the ground towards your buttocks. Use your hand to grab your ankle from behind, keeping your knees close together.
2. Feel the stretch in the front of your thigh – that's your quadriceps working their magic!
3. Hold this position for 20-30 seconds while maintaining good posture. Keep your chest up and shoulders relaxed.
4. Remember to breathe deeply and calmly throughout the stretch.
5. Slowly release your foot and return it to the ground.
6. Repeat the same process with your left leg.

Key Points

- Gradually increase the duration of the stretch as your flexibility improves.
- Keep your knees close together to maximize the stretch on your quadriceps.
- Maintain a straight posture with your chest up and shoulders relaxed.
- Always perform this stretch on both legs to ensure balance and symmetry.

Common Mistakes to Avoid

- Don't hurry through this exercise. A proper stretch takes time, so be patient, and you'll reap the benefits.
- While it's essential to challenge yourself, don't push your body too hard. Pain is not the goal here; a gentle stretch is.
- Keep that back straight! Slumping or hunching over takes away from the effectiveness of the stretch.
- Inhale and exhale deeply throughout the stretch to keep your body relaxed and oxygenated.
- Remember, it's crucial to stretch both legs to maintain balance in your body.

Butterfly Stretch

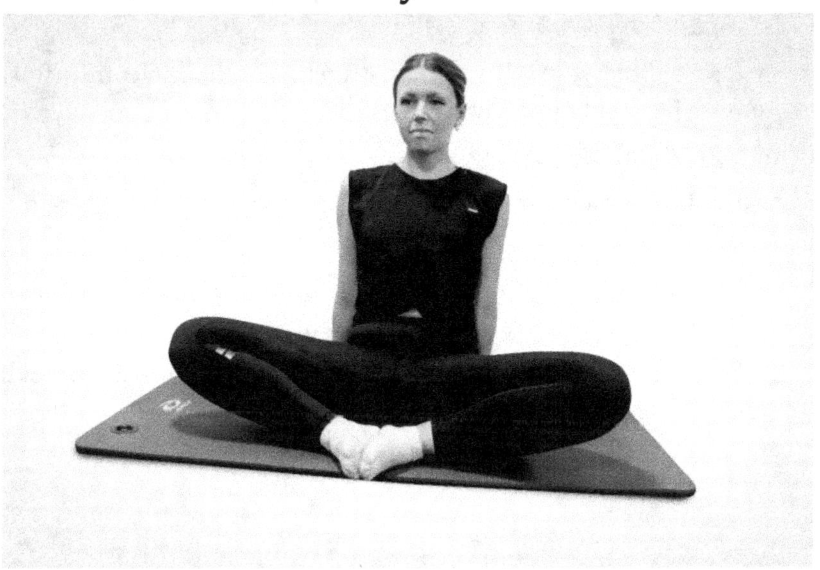

The Butterfly Stretch is like a soothing balm for your muscles. It targets your core and inner thighs – even giving your lower back some love! Practice it regularly, and you'll start to notice improved flexibility and less tension in your lower body.

The Setup

Find a comfortable spot on the floor or a yoga mat. Sit up tall with your back straight and your legs extended in front of you.

The Execution

Now, here comes the fun part!

1. Bend your knees outward like butterfly wings, bringing the soles of your feet together.

2. Hold your feet with your hands and gently pull them in towards your pelvis. Imagine your knees are trying to touch the floor.

3. Take a deep breath, and as you exhale, slowly lean forward from your hips while keeping your back straight. Feel that wonderful stretch in your inner thighs and groin area? That's the magic happening!

Key Points

- Remember to take slow, deep breaths as you lean forward. It'll help you relax into the stretch.

- This stretch isn't just about your legs. Feel your core muscles engage as you maintain good posture. It's like a double whammy for your midsection!

- Don't force yourself into the stretch. Gradually lean forward as your flexibility improves over time.

Common Mistakes to Avoid

- Keep that back straight! Avoid hunching over; it can strain your lower back.

- Be kind to your knees. Don't push them too hard towards the floor; work within your comfort zone.

- Breathing is your best friend. Don't forget to inhale and exhale; it'll make the stretch more effective.

Chapter 8: Advanced Core Techniques

It's essential to kick things off with a cautionary note: Before seniors dive into more advanced exercises, they must master the basics. Building a strong foundation in movement is like constructing a sturdy house – it ensures safety and stability throughout the journey to a healthier, more active life.

Before you dive into the exciting world of core exercises, there's an essential step you can't afford to skip – the warm-up! Warming up may sound like a mundane task, but it's your secret weapon for ensuring a safe and effective core workout. So, let's unravel the mysteries of warming up in a way that'll get you pumped and ready to go.

First things first, why should you bother with a warm-up? Well, think of your muscles and joints as a rubber band. When it's cold, the rubber band can snap easily. But when it's warm, it's stretchy and flexible. Your body's no different! Warming up increases blood flow, raises your body temperature, and makes your muscles and joints more pliable. This not only reduces the risk of injury but also enhances the overall performance of your core exercises.

Getting Started

Alright, let's get started with a simple yet effective warm-up routine tailored for seniors. Remember, it's not about pushing your limits right from the get-go; it's about easing into your workout gradually.

Gentle Aerobic Activity

Begin with 5-10 minutes of low-impact aerobic activity. You can choose activities like brisk walking, stationary cycling, or even gentle dancing. The idea is to get your heart rate up and start breaking a sweat. This will kickstart the blood flow to your muscles and lubricate your joints.

Joint Mobility Exercises

Next up, focus on your joints. Perform gentle joint mobility exercises to improve flexibility and reduce stiffness. Rotate your wrists, ankles, shoulders, and hips. Do some neck rolls and gentle head tilts from side to side. Move your joints through their full range of motion without forcing any movements.

Dynamic Stretches

Dynamic stretches are like a mini workout for your muscles while preparing them for action. Try leg swings, arm circles, or torso twists. These movements engage your muscles and gradually increase their flexibility.

Breathing Exercises

Don't forget to breathe! Take a few moments to practice deep, mindful breathing. Inhale slowly through your nose, expanding your chest and abdomen, then exhale fully through your mouth. This helps oxygenate your muscles and calms your mind for a focused workout.

Core-Specific Warm-Up

Before diving into the core exercises, it's wise to target the very muscles you're about to work on. Perform some light, core-specific warm-up exercises. Try gentle pelvic tilts, cat-cow stretches, or modified planks. These movements activate your core muscles and get them ready for the main event.

Tips for a Safe Warm-Up

Now that you know what to do, here are some tips to make your warm-up even safer and more effective:

- Start Slow: Don't rush through your warm-up. Take your time and listen to your body.

- Pain-Free Zone: Warm-up exercises should never cause pain. If something hurts, stop immediately.

- Gradual Progression: As you become more accustomed to your routine, you can gradually increase the intensity and duration of your warm-up.

- Stay Hydrated: Sip some water before and during your warm-up to stay hydrated.

- Proper Attire: Wear comfortable, breathable clothing and supportive shoes.

- Stay Consistent: Make warming up a non-negotiable part of your core workout routine.

When it comes to core exercises for seniors, we've covered the basics that help improve stability and strength. But now, let's take things up a notch and delve into some more exciting and intricate moves to give your core a real workout.

Remember, always consult with your healthcare provider before starting any new exercise routine, especially if you have underlying health conditions.

Pilates-inspired Core Engagements

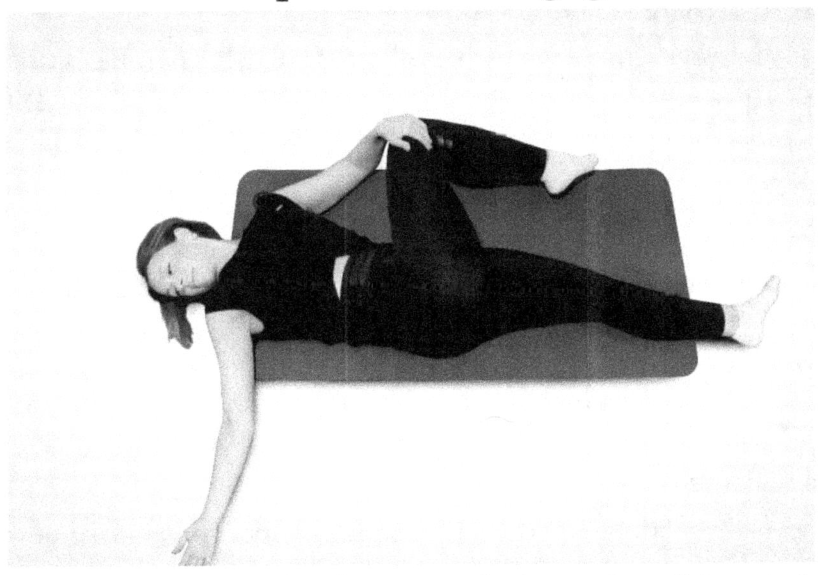

Pilates, a fitness regimen that focuses on the integration of the mind and body, has garnered significant acclaim due to its capacity to enhance core strength while simultaneously enhancing flexibility and balance. These exercises may appear daunting at first, but with patience and persistence, they can be adapted to suit various fitness levels. Let's start with some Pilates-inspired Core Engagements that will help you build a rock-solid core.

Before we dive into the specifics, let's get you set up for success. Find a comfortable, flat surface to lay down on, preferably a yoga mat or a soft carpet. Wear loose, breathable clothing, and keep a water bottle nearby to stay hydrated. Remember, safety comes first!

The Setup

- Begin by lying on your back with your legs extended straight and your arms resting by your sides, palms facing down. Ensure that your spine is in a neutral position, with your natural lower back curve maintained.

- If you have lower back issues, consider bending your knees with your feet flat on the floor for added support. This modification can reduce strain on the lower back.

- Gently lift your head and neck off the ground, keeping your chin slightly tucked. This is the starting position for your upper body.

The Execution

1. Lift your arms a few inches off the ground, keeping them straight. Begin to pulse them up and down, taking quick, controlled breaths. Inhale for five arm pulses, and exhale for five pulses. Keep your core engaged throughout.

2. The rhythmic breathing is crucial to The Hundred. It helps oxygenate your body and engage your core muscles effectively. Imagine filling your lungs with air like a balloon on the inhale and squeezing out the air on the exhale.

3. Aim to complete 100 arm pulses while maintaining the breathing pattern. This exercise may take a while to build up to, so start with a lower number and work your way up gradually.

Key Points

- The Hundred primarily targets your abdominal muscles. Ensure that you're engaging them throughout the exercise to maximize its effectiveness.

- Maintain a steady and controlled pace with your arm pulses and breathing. Rushing through the exercise can lead to improper form.

- Avoid straining your neck by keeping it in line with your spine. If it becomes uncomfortable, lower your head and neck to the ground briefly.

Common Mistakes to Avoid

- Be cautious not to arch your lower back excessively. This can strain your spine. If you feel this is happening, try the modified version with bent knees.

- Remember, proper breathing is crucial. Holding your breath can lead to dizziness and reduce the effectiveness of the exercise.

- Maintain smooth, controlled arm pulses. Avoid jerking or swinging your arms, as this can strain your shoulders and detract from the core workout.

- If you're a beginner or have physical limitations, don't be afraid to modify The Hundred to suit your needs. Gradually work your way up to the full exercise.

Progression Steps

- Increase the number of arm pulses gradually. Start with 10 and work your way up to 100 as you build strength and endurance.

- Extend your leg position: To add more challenge, lift your legs off the ground, keeping them straight. This engages your lower abdominals and adds a new dimension to the exercise.

- Explore variations: There are numerous adaptations of The Hundred, such as using props like resistance bands or small hand weights to increase resistance.

Remember, your fitness journey is a personal one. Listen to your body, and if you experience any pain or discomfort, consult with a healthcare professional before continuing. The Hundred can be a powerful tool in your quest for a stronger core, but safety and proper form should always come first.

Side Planks with Leg Raises

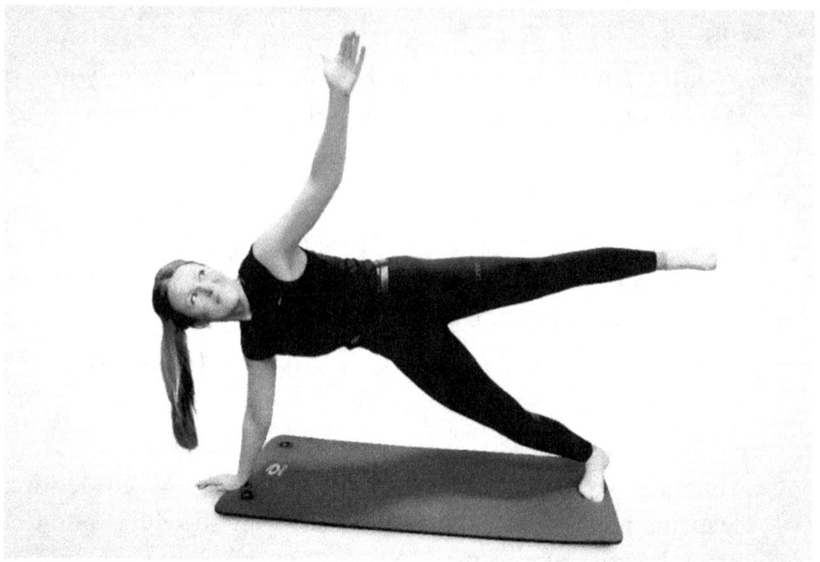

Side Planks with Leg Raises are your secret weapon, and they're not as intimidating as they might sound. In fact, they're perfect for seniors looking to add a dash of excitement to their workout routine.

The Setup

- First things first, let's set the stage for the Side Planks with Leg Raises exercise. Find a comfortable and flat surface, preferably a yoga mat or a carpeted area, where you can stretch out without slipping. Remember, safety is our top priority here, so choose a spot where you feel secure.

- Start by lying on your side with your legs fully extended. Your elbow should be directly beneath your shoulder, forming a 90-degree angle.

- Place your top hand on your hip or extend it upward toward the ceiling for added stability and balance.

- Engage your core muscles by imagining you're pulling your belly button towards your spine. This is your starting position.

The Execution

1. Lift your hips off the ground, keeping your body in a straight line from your head to your heels. You should be supporting your weight on your forearm and the side of your bottom foot.

2. Once you're in a stable side plank position, it's leg-raising time! Slowly lift your top leg as high as you comfortably can while maintaining your balance. Keep your toes pointed forward to ensure proper form.

3. Lower your leg back down to meet the other one, but don't let it touch the ground. Repeat this leg raise motion for your desired number of repetitions.

Key Points

- Keep your core engaged throughout the exercise. This helps protect your lower back and ensures you're getting the most out of the workout.

- Maintain proper alignment. Your body should form a straight line from head to heels while in the side plank position.

- Focus on controlled movements. Don't rush through the leg raises; instead, perform them slowly and with intention.

- Breathe! Inhale deeply through your nose as you prepare, and exhale through your mouth as you lift your leg.

- Listen to your body. If you experience pain or discomfort, stop immediately and consult with a healthcare professional.

Common Mistakes to Avoid

- It's crucial to maintain that straight line from head to heels. Avoid letting your hips sag towards the ground.

- While lifting your leg, don't go beyond your comfortable range of motion. Overextension can lead to strain or injury.

- Breathing is an essential part of any exercise. Don't hold your breath during Side Planks with Leg Raises; it can lead to dizziness and discomfort.

- Ensure your body is adequately warmed up before attempting this exercise. Cold muscles are more prone to injury.

Progression Steps and Modifications

- Start with a few reps and gradually work your way up to more. Aim for 10-15 raises per side to begin with.

- Extend the duration of your side plank hold to build endurance. Begin with 15-20 seconds and progress from there.

- For added resistance, you can strap on some ankle weights while performing leg raises. Start with light weights and increase gradually.

- If maintaining the side plank position is challenging, use a sturdy chair or wall for support until you build enough strength.

Remember, be patient with yourself, and don't be discouraged if you can't perform these exercises perfectly right away. Every step counts toward a stronger, healthier you. Keep pushing yourself gently, and always prioritize safety over intensity. You've got this!

Russian Twists

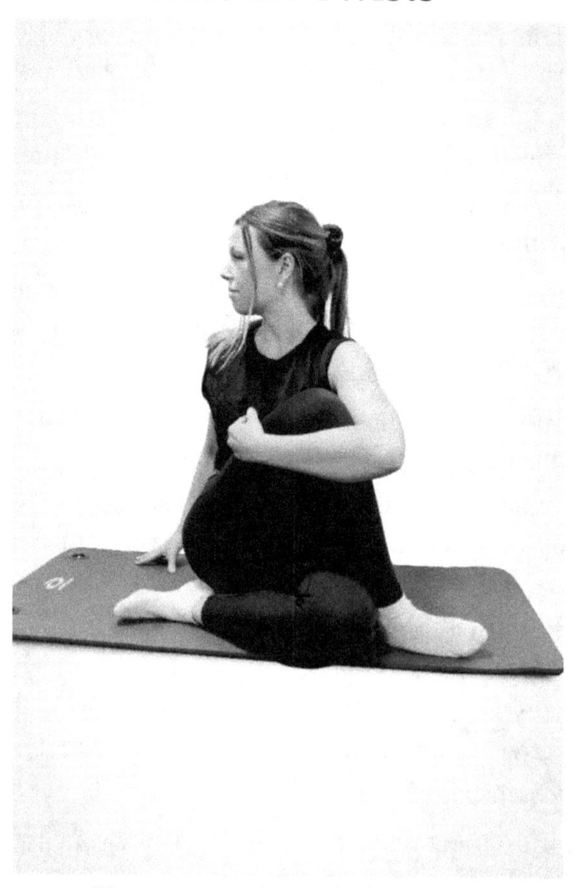

Russian Twists are like a secret handshake among fitness enthusiasts. They not only help sculpt your core but also enhance your balance and posture. So, seniors, get ready to feel your core come alive like never before!

The Setup

- Begin by choosing a quiet and comfortable place to practice your Russian Twists. It could be in your living room, garden, or even at the gym.

- Next, grab a sturdy chair or lay down a yoga mat. This will provide you with the support you need during the exercise.

The Execution

1. Start by sitting on the chair or mat with your back straight and shoulders relaxed. Bend your knees and keep your feet flat on the ground.

2. Bring your hands together in front of you, palms touching.

3. Engage your core muscles by pulling your navel toward your spine. This will create a stable base for the exercise.

4. Slowly twist your upper body to the right, keeping your hips square. Imagine you're trying to touch your right elbow to the back of the chair or mat.

5. After twisting to the right, come back to the center with control. Make sure to maintain good posture throughout the movement.

6. Repeat the twist, this time to the left side, aiming to touch your left elbow to the back of the chair or mat.

7. Bring your upper body back to the center position.

Key Points

- Focus on controlled movements. Don't rush through the twists; instead, maintain a steady and deliberate pace.

- Remember to breathe steadily. Inhale as you return to the center and exhale as you twist.

- Your feet should remain flat on the ground throughout the exercise to maintain balance and stability.

- Sit up straight, and keep your shoulders relaxed. Imagine a string pulling you up from the top of your head.

Common Mistakes to Avoid

- Avoid over-rotating your upper body; this can strain your back.

- Don't rush through the twists; this can lead to a loss of form and effectiveness.

- Remember to engage your core muscles continuously; it's the powerhouse behind this exercise.

- Keep the breath flowing naturally. Holding your breath can lead to dizziness.

Progression Steps

- Hold a light dumbbell, water bottle, or a small household item to increase resistance.

- Lift your feet slightly off the ground while maintaining good form. This intensifies the exercise.

- Gradually increase the number of twists you perform in each set.

- As you get more comfortable, you can slightly increase the speed of your twists while still maintaining control.

Modifications

- If twisting all the way is too tough, limit your range of motion. Twist just a little to the sides until you build more strength.

- Sit on a cushion or pillow to elevate your hips, making the exercise more manageable.

- Keep your feet flat, but bend your knees less to make the twists less intense.

Remember, the most important thing is to listen to your body. If something doesn't feel right or causes discomfort, adjust accordingly. Safety and comfort should always come first.

So, let's make Russian Twists your new core-building buddies. Strengthening your core not only enhances your daily activities but also keeps you feeling vibrant and confident. Happy twisting, and keep rocking that strong core!

Reverse Planks

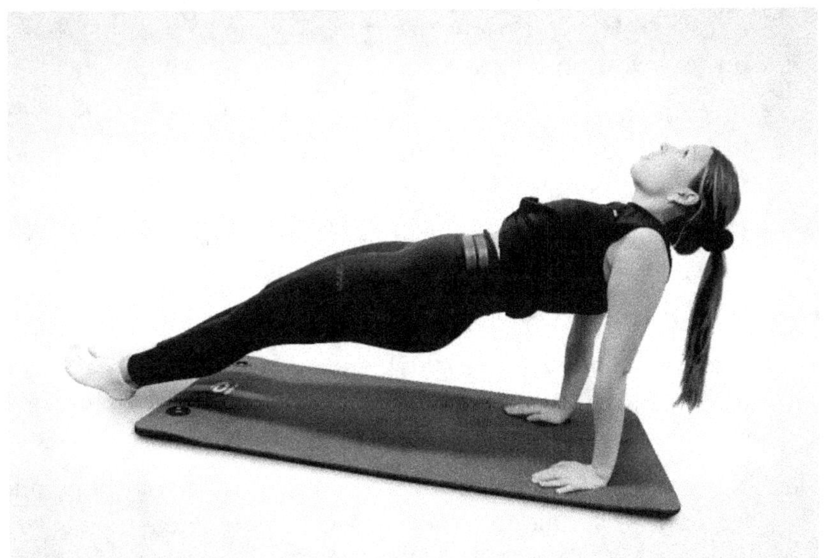

Reverse Planks are your ticket to building a rock-solid midsection while having some fun along the way. Don't be intimidated by the word "reverse" – we're here to guide you through this fantastic exercise.

The Setup

Grab a comfortable mat or find a smooth, non-slip surface. Sit down with your legs extended straight in front of you, hip-width apart. Place your hands behind your hips, fingers pointing toward your feet, and press them firmly into the ground. Make sure your shoulders are relaxed and your chest is open. Keep your neck in a neutral position, looking forward.

The Execution

1. Lift your hips off the ground while keeping your legs straight.
2. Your body should form a straight line from head to heels.
3. Engage your core muscles to provide assistance for the back.
4. Imagine pushing your chest upward and slightly forward while lengthening your neck.
5. Hold this position for a few breaths or as long as you feel comfortable.

Key Points

- The key to a successful Reverse Plank is engaging your core muscles. This not only strengthens your midsection but also protects your lower back.

- Imagine pushing your chest forward and upward to create a beautiful arch in your upper back. This not only looks impressive but also helps improve posture.

- Don't forget to breathe! Inhale and exhale deeply to stay relaxed and maintain focus.

Common Mistakes to Avoid

- The most common mistake is not engaging the core. This puts unnecessary strain on your lower back and takes away the core-strengthening benefits.

- Keep those shoulders away from your ears! Avoid hunching or letting your shoulders droop to prevent shoulder strain.

- Maintain a neutral neck position. Avoid looking up or down excessively, as this can strain your neck.

Progression Steps

- Start with short holds, maybe 10-15 seconds, and gradually increase the duration as your strength improves.

- Once you're comfortable with the basic Reverse Plank, challenge yourself by lifting one leg at a time while maintaining the plank position.

- Take it up a notch by transitioning into a single-leg Reverse Plank. Lift one leg and hold it straight up for a few seconds before switching to the other.

- For an extra challenge, try placing your feet on an elevated surface like a step or a sturdy bench. This increases the range of motion and intensifies the workout.

Bird-Dog with Stability Challenges

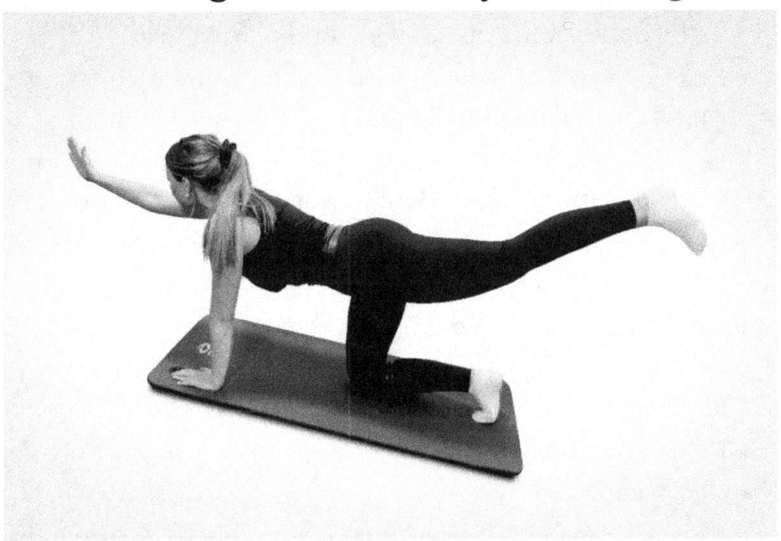

In this exciting part of our journey, we're diving into the fantastic world of Bird-Dog with Stability Challenges exercises! These moves are like the secret ingredients to baking a cake - they're the building blocks for a stronger core that'll leave you feeling more robust and energetic than ever before.

The Setup

To get started, find a comfy spot on the floor or a yoga mat. Get on all fours, with your hands directly under your shoulders and your knees under your hips. Engage that core by pulling your belly button towards your spine. Now, make sure your neck and spine are in a nice, neutral position. You're all set up and ready to soar!

The Execution

1. Extend your right arm forward and your left leg back at the same time. Imagine you're reaching out for something tasty in front of you and something fun to chase behind you.

2. Hold that position for a few seconds, then gently lower your arm and leg back to the starting position.

3. Now, switch to the left arm and right leg.

4. Keep alternating like you're dancing to your favorite tune. Do 10-15 reps for each side, and you'll be on your way to a stronger core.

Key Points

- Keep your hips level with the ground. Don't let one hip sneak up higher than the other - it's a level playing field!

- Engage your core throughout the movement. Imagine you're zipping up a tight pair of pants.

- Breathe steadily. Inhale as you reach out, exhale as you return to the starting position. Breathing is your secret power.

- Don't rush! Slow and steady wins the race here. Make every movement count.

Common Mistakes to Avoid

- Avoid leaning to one side when you extend your arm and leg. It's all about balance, not a tilt-a-whirl!

- Keep that back nice and flat. Don't arch it like a cat stretching after a nap.

- Keep your head in line with your spine. No need to look at the ceiling or the floor - it's all happening right in front of you.

Progression Steps

You can increase the challenge by using a stability ball or a foam roller. Place the ball or roller under your extended arm and leg. This adds a wobbly element that'll really fire up those core muscles.

Modifications

If you're just starting out or have some physical limitations, no worries! You can modify this exercise to fit your needs. Instead of extending your arm and leg all the way, try lifting them just a few inches off the ground. It's like Bird-Dog Lite! You'll still feel the benefits without the full-blown challenge.

If you have any pre-existing health conditions or concerns, it's a good idea to consult with a healthcare professional or fitness expert before diving into advanced exercises. Your safety and well-being are our top priorities!

Chapter 9: Make Core Exercise Your Lifestyle

Are you tired of the same old fitness routines that seem more like chores than enjoyable activities? Well, it's time to shake things up and make core exercise a vibrant part of your lifestyle. Forget about those endless hours on the treadmill or the monotonous reps at the gym. Core exercise is about more than just getting a six-pack; it's about enhancing your overall health, posture, and strength while having fun along the way.

Strength That Lasts a Lifetime: When you engage your core regularly, you're building a strong foundation for your entire body. It's not just about getting those washboard abs; it's about having the strength to lift your kids, carry groceries, or even prevent back pain as you age. Core strength is your ticket to a lifetime of physical resilience.

Effortless Posture: Slouching? Say goodbye to it! A strong core naturally pulls you into good posture. No more hunching over your desk or feeling like the Hunchback of Notre Dame. With a strong core, you'll stand tall and proud, exuding confidence.

Injury Prevention: Ever rolled your ankle or hurt your back doing mundane tasks? A stable core acts like your body's armor. It protects you from those annoying everyday injuries by providing stability and balance. You become less accident-prone and more agile in your movements.

Aging Gracefully: We all want to age like fine wine, right? Consistent core engagement helps you maintain mobility as the years roll by. Forget about shuffling around; you'll be dancing your way into your golden years.

Boosted Metabolism: Want to rev up your metabolism without downing questionable supplements? A strong core does just that! It keeps your internal engine running smoothly, helping you burn more calories even at rest. It's like having a perpetual fat-burning furnace inside you.

Rock-Solid Confidence: Confidence isn't just about how you look; it's about how you feel. When you're strong at your core, you radiate confidence. You'll feel more self-assured in social situations, at work, and even when tackling new challenges.

Pain-Free Living: Tired of those nagging aches and pains? Strengthening your core can often alleviate or even eliminate chronic pain, especially in the lower back. Say goodbye to that constant ache and hello to pain-free living.

Enhanced Sports Performance: Whether you're a weekend warrior or a seasoned athlete, a strong core is your secret weapon. It improves your balance, power, and agility, giving you an edge in your favorite sports and activities.

Better Digestion: Believe it or not, a healthy core can aid digestion. It supports your organs and helps them function optimally. Say goodbye to bloating and indigestion.

Mental Toughness: The discipline required for consistent core engagement spills over into other areas of your life. You'll find yourself more focused, determined, and ready to conquer challenges.

So, how can you make core exercise a lifestyle? Start small and build up gradually. Incorporate core exercises into your daily routine. Even a few minutes each day can make a big difference over time. You don't need fancy equipment; bodyweight exercises like planks, leg raises, and Russian twists can do wonders.

Consistency is key

Consistency is absolutely crucial when it comes to making core exercise a lifestyle. Imagine it like this: just as you wouldn't skip brushing your teeth, you shouldn't skip engaging your core. It needs to become as non-negotiable as your daily dental routine. The good news is you don't have to resort to tedious workouts that feel like a chore. There are plenty of enjoyable activities that can help you strengthen your core while having fun.

One fantastic option is yoga. The serene flow of yoga not only helps you find inner peace but also engages your core muscles in a subtle yet effective way. It's a holistic practice that combines stretching, balance, and mindfulness, making it an ideal choice for those who want to make core engagement a regular part of their lives. Plus, there's a multitude of yoga styles to choose from, so you can find the one that best suits your preferences.

Pilates is another exciting path to core strength. This low-impact exercise method focuses on precision and controlled movements, all of which target your core muscles. Pilates workouts can vary in intensity, making them suitable for people of all fitness levels. The best part? It never gets boring, thanks to the diverse range of exercises and equipment available, from mat-based routines to reformer machines.

If you're someone who loves to dance, you're in luck! Dancing is not just a way to express yourself; it's also a fantastic core workout in disguise. Whether you're into salsa, hip-hop, or ballroom dancing, you'll find that moving to the rhythm engages your core muscles naturally. It's a great way to get your heart pumping while having a blast on the dance floor. So, why not join a dance class or simply put on your favorite tunes and let loose at home?

To ensure consistency in your core exercise journey, consider enlisting a workout buddy or hiring a personal trainer. Having a workout buddy can turn your core workouts into social events. It adds an element of accountability and motivation to your routine. You're less likely to skip a session when you know someone is counting on you. Plus, it's a fantastic way to bond with a friend or family member while working towards your fitness goals together.

If you prefer a more personalized approach, a certified trainer can be your guiding light. They can create a customized core workout plan tailored to your specific needs and goals. A trainer also provides expert guidance, ensuring you perform exercises correctly and safely. Their expertise can help you avoid common mistakes that may lead to injury or hinder your progress.

Now, let's talk about an essential aspect of core exercise: listening to your body. While consistency is key, it's equally important to recognize when your body needs a break or when something doesn't feel quite right. Pain during an exercise is a red flag that should never be ignored. If you experience pain, stop immediately and seek guidance from a fitness professional.

Remember, safety should always be your top priority. Pushing through pain can lead to injuries that set you back on your fitness journey. Instead, consult with a fitness expert who can assess your form, suggest modifications, or recommend alternative exercises that are safer for your body. Your long-term health and well-being depend on taking care of yourself during your core workouts.

Setting a Schedule

Life gets hectic, and sometimes, staying consistent with core exercises can be a real challenge. But if you want to make core exercise a natural part of your daily routine, *consistency is your golden ticket.* Think of setting a schedule as laying the foundation for a strong and healthy lifestyle. It's like planting the seeds that will grow into a robust tree of core strength. A schedule provides structure and turns exercise from an occasional chore into a habit that sticks.

Imagine waking up each morning with a clear plan in your mind for when and how you'll engage those core muscles. It becomes as automatic as brushing your teeth or sipping your morning coffee. So, let's dive into some practical strategies to make setting and sticking to your core exercise schedule a breeze.

Start Small, Grow Steadily

Attempting to revolutionize your entire daily routine all at once is a recipe for burnout and frustration. Instead, adopt a more measured approach by commencing with manageable, small steps. Allocate just a few minutes each day to engage in core exercises, and incrementally extend this duration as your strength and endurance show signs of enhancement. In the initial stages, prioritize consistency over intensity.

Embarking on a journey of self-improvement necessitates a patient and sustainable approach. By starting small and growing steadily, you're setting yourself up for success, allowing your body and mind to adapt and thrive over time. This incremental method ensures that you don't overwhelm yourself, increasing the likelihood of long-term adherence to your fitness goals. Remember, the tortoise's slow and steady pace ultimately won the race, and your path to a healthier lifestyle can follow the same principle.

Find Your Golden Hours

One essential step in achieving your fitness goals is to pinpoint the specific moments of the day when your energy and motivation are at their peak. Is it the early hours of the morning when the world is still waking up? Perhaps it's during your midday break when you have a moment to refresh and recharge. Alternatively, you might find that your inner fire blazes brightest in the tranquil hours of the evening. Whatever your golden hours may be, recognizing and harnessing them is crucial for maintaining a consistent exercise routine that yields lasting results.

Tailoring your core exercise schedule to align with your personal peak performance times can make a world of difference in your fitness journey. Here's how it works:

- Morning Energizers: If you're a morning person, seize the day by scheduling your workouts during the early hours. Morning exercise can kickstart your metabolism, boost your mood, and provide a sense of accomplishment that sets a positive tone for the rest of your day.

- Midday Revival: If your motivation tends to surge during your lunch break, consider making this your designated exercise time. It's a great way to break up the workday, alleviate stress, and ensure you stay energized and focused for the afternoon tasks ahead.

- Evening Warriors: For those who come alive in the evening, nighttime workouts can be the perfect way to unwind, release pent-up energy, and decompress after a busy day. Just be mindful of not exercising too close to bedtime, as it may interfere with your sleep.

Calendar Commitment

When it comes to ensuring your fitness routine stays on track, one powerful strategy is to integrate it seamlessly into your daily schedule. To do this effectively, take out your calendar, whether it's a digital app on your phone or a physical planner, and allocate specific time slots for your core workout sessions. Treat these appointments with the same level of commitment and importance as you would for any other crucial event in your life, be it a work meeting, a doctor's appointment, or a dinner reservation.

By visually marking these dedicated time slots in your calendar, you accomplish two significant things. First, it sends a clear message to yourself that your health and fitness are non-negotiable priorities in your life. Second, it serves as a constant and visual reminder of your commitment to your core workout routine, making it less likely for you to forget or procrastinate.

Mix It Up

Embracing variety in your fitness regimen can truly transform your core exercise routine into a dynamic and exciting endeavor. The age-old adage, "variety is the spice of life," couldn't be more apt when it comes to sculpting your core muscles and achieving lasting fitness results. By infusing your workouts with a diverse array of exercises, such as planks, leg raises, and bicycle crunches, you can elevate your core training to a whole new level.

The beauty of incorporating a mix of exercises is that it injects a sense of novelty and excitement into your workouts. This, in turn, serves as a powerful antidote to boredom, a common nemesis that can thwart your fitness progress. When you constantly challenge your body with different movements, you not only prevent monotony but also keep your mind engaged and motivated throughout your fitness journey.

Buddy System

Embracing a fitness journey becomes a more enjoyable and productive endeavor when you involve a close friend or family member in the process. This dynamic duo, known as the "buddy system," offers a plethora of benefits that extend beyond just breaking a sweat together. This approach to fitness is a powerful synergy of camaraderie, mutual motivation, and accountability.

First and foremost, having a workout partner transforms exercise routines into memorable and fun experiences. The shared laughter, encouragement, and friendly competition create an engaging atmosphere that helps combat the monotony of repetitive workouts. Those moments of joy and shared accomplishments can make each session something to look forward to, making it easier to stay consistent and committed to your fitness goals.

Reward Yourself

Harnessing the power of positive reinforcement can be a game-changer when it comes to cultivating a consistent core exercise habit. It's essential to acknowledge and celebrate your achievements, no matter how small they may seem. After successfully completing a planned workout session, consider indulging in a well-deserved treat that not only serves as a motivational pat on the back but also adds an element of joy to your fitness journey. Here are some delightful ideas to help you reward yourself and keep the motivation flowing:

- Nutrient-Packed Smoothie Delight: Blend up a scrumptious and nutritious smoothie packed with your favorite fruits, vegetables, and a scoop of protein powder. This delicious concoction not only replenishes your energy but also aids in muscle recovery.

- Pampering Bath Experience: Treat yourself to a rejuvenating bath filled with Epsom salts and aromatic essential oils. This soothing soak not only relaxes your tired muscles but also provides a serene moment to unwind and reflect on your fitness progress.

- Entertainment Escape: Dive into the world of entertainment by watching your all-time favorite TV show, movie, or series. This not only provides a well-deserved break but also keeps you motivated as you eagerly anticipate your next viewing session as a reward.

Be Flexible

In the ever-changing landscape of life, it's crucial to embrace the concept of flexibility. Unexpected twists and turns are inevitable, and your meticulously planned schedule may occasionally require adjustments. This is not only acceptable but often necessary for maintaining a healthy and sustainable routine. The essential aspect is not to abandon your habits altogether. When you encounter a disruption, view it as an opportunity to adapt and recalibrate.

If you happen to miss a scheduled session, rather than chastising yourself, opt for a more constructive approach. Reschedule the missed activity for a later time or day, allowing yourself the chance to make up for it. Remember that even the most dedicated individuals encounter hiccups in their routines, so there's no need to be overly critical.

Track Your Progress

One of the keys to a successful core exercise routine is to track your progress diligently. You can do this by maintaining a journal dedicated to your fitness journey or by utilizing a fitness app tailored to your needs.

Keeping a record of your core exercise sessions is not just a mundane task; it's a powerful tool that can fuel your motivation and enhance your commitment to achieving your fitness goals.

Imagine your fitness journal or app as a virtual garden where you carefully plant the seeds of your efforts during each core exercise session. Every entry represents a seed, and as you water and nurture them with your dedication, you'll soon witness the remarkable growth in your strength and endurance. It's akin to watching a tree you planted grow taller each day, a tangible and awe-inspiring testament to your hard work and dedication.

Visual Reminders

In the pursuit of maintaining a steadfast commitment to your core exercise regimen, it can be immensely beneficial to incorporate visual reminders strategically within your living space. These visual cues not only serve as a constant source of motivation but also play a pivotal role in keeping your fitness objectives at the forefront of your daily routine.

Sticky notes are a simple yet highly effective tool for keeping your core exercise goals on track. Consider placing colorful Post-It notes in prominent locations around your home, such as on your bathroom mirror, the refrigerator door, or your workspace. Write down brief motivational messages or specific workout targets to keep yourself focused and driven throughout the day.

Surrounding yourself with motivational quotes can provide a daily dose of encouragement. Select inspiring quotes that resonate with your fitness aspirations and create visually appealing displays. Frame them or use decorative calligraphy to make them visually striking, then position them in areas where you spend a significant amount of time, such as your bedroom or kitchen.

Celebrate Milestones

Setting milestones is an essential aspect of any journey towards self-improvement and success. These checkpoints serve as guiding lights, helping you stay on track and measure your progress. However, achieving these milestones isn't just about reaching the destination; it's also about enjoying the journey itself. By acknowledging your accomplishments, whether they are big or small, you can infuse your path with motivation, dedication, and a sense of fulfillment.

Imagine you're on a fitness journey. You've committed to working out regularly, and today, you've managed to hold a challenging plank position for an extra 10 seconds. It may not seem like a monumental achievement, but it's a noteworthy step forward in your fitness goals. By celebrating this accomplishment, you are reinforcing your commitment to your well-being.

Similarly, in various aspects of life, you might set goals such as completing a certain number of repetitions at work, in your studies, or in your personal projects. These goals are like stepping stones that lead you toward your ultimate objectives. Recognizing and celebrating your progress along the way can have a profound impact on your mindset and motivation.

Celebrating milestones doesn't necessarily mean throwing a grand party for every achievement. It can be as simple as giving yourself a pat on the back, treating yourself to a small indulgence, or sharing your success with a friend or family member. The key is to acknowledge the effort and dedication you've put in and to use these moments of celebration as fuel to keep moving forward.

The Power of Exercise Diaries

Exercise diaries are like your personal fitness journal. They help you track your progress, set goals, and stay accountable. Think of them as your exercise BFF. Here's how to make the most of them:

Recording Your Workouts: First things first, grab your exercise diary and jot down your core exercises. Note the number of reps you did and how long you sweated it out during each session. This simple act of recording your efforts creates a visual record of your dedication. It's like a high-five from your past self, reminding you to keep going and stay on track.

Setting Realistic Goals: Now, let's talk about goals! Your exercise diary is the perfect place to set and track your fitness aspirations. These goals should be like stepping stones, not towering mountains. Whether it's increasing your plank-holding endurance by an extra 10 seconds or pushing yourself to do a few more sit-ups each day, these mini-milestones will keep the fire of inspiration burning bright.

Planning Ahead: Failing to plan is planning to fail, they say, and it couldn't be truer in the world of core exercise. Use your exercise diary to map out your fitness journey. Schedule your core workouts in advance, just like you would any other important appointment. Be specific with your timings. When you have a set time to exercise, it becomes a commitment, not just an idea floating in your mind. This makes it harder to skip a session because, hey, you wouldn't bail on a meeting with your boss, right?

But wait, there's more to the magic of exercise diaries!

They Boost Your Accountability: Imagine having a workout buddy who never lets you skip a session. That's what an exercise diary does for you. It holds you accountable. When you see those empty spaces in your diary, it's a nudge, a gentle reminder that you've got a date with your mat or weights. It's like having a personal trainer and a motivational speaker rolled into one.

They Show Patterns: As you fill in your exercise diary over time, you'll start noticing patterns. Maybe you're more motivated to work out in the mornings or on weekends. Perhaps you see a dip in your enthusiasm during stressful weeks. These insights help you tailor your fitness routine to your unique rhythm, ensuring you stay engaged and consistent.

They Build Confidence: Remember the first time you successfully held a plank for 30 seconds or completed a set of challenging exercises? Those moments are golden, and your exercise diary captures them all. Flipping through those pages filled with your achievements can be a massive confidence booster. It's like having a journal of your superhero moments, reminding you that you're capable of incredible feats.

They Are a Source of Inspiration: On days when motivation seems to have taken a vacation, your exercise diary becomes your source of inspiration. It's a tangible record of your progress, a testament to your hard work. Whenever doubt creeps in, a quick glance at your past accomplishments can reignite the spark of determination within you.

They Foster Discipline: Constantly filling in your exercise diary requires discipline. It instills a sense of order in your fitness routine, helping you stay focused on your goals. Just like brushing your teeth or having your morning coffee, it becomes a non-negotiable part of your daily life.

They Keep You Committed: Life can get busy, and distractions are everywhere. But your exercise diary serves as a constant reminder of your commitment to a healthier you. When you feel like slacking off, it whispers, "You've got this!" and pushes you to keep going.

Smartphone Reminders: Your Workout Buddy

In today's fast-paced digital world, where our smartphones are practically an extension of our hands, it's time to harness the power of these pocket-sized marvels to make core exercise an integral part of your daily lifestyle. Say goodbye to mundane reminders and hello to an engaging and effective fitness routine with these tips on how to use smartphone reminders to your advantage:

Set Daily Alarms: Let's start with the basics. The first step to making core exercise a lifestyle is to schedule daily alarms or notifications on your smartphone. Think of these alarms as your personal fitness concierge, always ready to remind you to get moving. Whether you prefer a gentle morning reminder to kickstart your day or a midday nudge to break up your work routine, your phone can be your reliable workout buddy. Consistency is vital, and these daily alarms will ensure that your core exercises become a non-negotiable part of your routine.

Customize Your Alerts: Now, let's add some flair to those reminders. Personalization is a powerful motivator, so why not customize your alerts with motivational messages? Instead of a plain "Time for your workout," try something like, "Time to work those abs!" It may seem simple, but these words can transform a mundane reminder into a mini pep talk. Your smartphone can become your very own cheerleader, pushing you to give your best effort with every core exercise session. So go ahead, get creative, and make those reminders resonate with your fitness journey.

Sync with Your Calendar: Efficiency is critical when it comes to balancing our busy lives with fitness goals. To ensure that your core exercises seamlessly fit into your daily routine, integrate your exercise schedule with your digital calendar. By syncing your workouts with your appointments, meetings, and other commitments, you can prioritize your fitness without the risk of double-booking or missing a session. This smart approach allows you to plan your day around your core routine, making it easier than ever to maintain your commitment to a healthy lifestyle.

Use Fitness Apps: In the vast world of smartphone applications, there's a treasure trove of fitness apps waiting for you. These apps not only offer workout plans tailored to your goals but also provide timely reminders to keep you on track. Many of these fitness apps come equipped with built-in timers and step-by-step tutorials to guide you through your core exercises. Whether you're a beginner looking to learn the ropes or a seasoned fitness enthusiast in search of a new challenge, these apps have you covered. With a variety of options at your fingertips, you can choose the one that suits your preferences and keeps you engaged in your core exercise journey.

Share Your Goals: Are you the type who thrives on social interaction and accountability? If so, consider sharing your workout goals and progress on social media. Your online community can serve as a source of motivation and support. Sharing your achievements, no matter how small, not only celebrates your progress but also inspires others on their fitness journeys. By making your fitness goals public, you create a sense of responsibility to stay consistent and achieve what you set out to do. Plus, the encouragement and feedback from friends and followers can be a powerful boost to your core exercise lifestyle.

Creating a Core Exercise Habit

If you're looking to make core exercise a part of your daily life, the key is to turn it into a habit. Experts say that it takes about 21 days to establish a routine, so don't get discouraged if it feels challenging at first. To help you stick with it, here are some tips that will make core exercise a natural part of your lifestyle.

Start Slow: The journey to a strong core begins with small steps. Instead of diving headfirst into intense workouts, start with a manageable routine. Begin with exercises that match your current fitness level. It's better to begin modestly and gradually increase the intensity and duration as your stamina improves. By doing so, you'll avoid burnout and the temptation to quit prematurely.

Find Joy in the Process: Exercise doesn't have to be a chore. Select core exercises that genuinely bring you joy. Whether it's the fluid movements of yoga, the precision of Pilates, or the rhythm of dancing, choosing an activity you love can make all the difference. When you have fun, you're more likely to look forward to your workouts and stay committed to your routine.

Track Your Progress: Keeping track of your core exercise journey is both motivating and enlightening. Create a workout journal or use a fitness app to record your workouts, sets, reps, and any improvements you notice. Tracking your progress allows you to see how far you've come, which can be a powerful motivator when faced with challenges. It also helps you identify areas where you might need to adjust your routine for better results.

Stay Flexible: While consistency is crucial, it's equally important to remain flexible. Life can throw unexpected curveballs, and there may be days when you can't stick to your planned workout schedule. Instead of feeling guilty or discouraged, adapt to the situation. Fit in a quick core exercise session when you have a spare moment, or simply accept that some days are meant for rest. The key is to maintain a long-term perspective and not let occasional setbacks derail your overall progress.

Educate Yourself: Knowledge is power, and understanding the benefits of core exercise can be a motivating factor. Research and learn about how core strength contributes to your overall health and well-being. When you appreciate the positive impact it has on your posture, balance, and even everyday activities, you'll be more inclined to prioritize core exercises in your daily life.

Stay Patient and Positive: Building a core exercise habit, like any habit, takes time. There will be days when you don't feel like working out or when you encounter challenges. During these moments, it's crucial to stay patient and maintain a positive mindset. Remember why you started this journey in the first place, and focus on the long-term benefits of a strong core. With persistence and a positive attitude, you can transform core exercise into a natural and enjoyable part of your lifestyle.

Chapter 10: Success Stories and Why They Matter

In a world filled with endless distractions and temptations, making core exercise a part of your daily life might sound like a daunting task. No worries; in this book, we've explored how you can turn core exercise into a lifestyle that's not only enjoyable but also incredibly rewarding.

Let's kick things off by delving into the fascinating world of motivation. Understanding why you want to make core exercise a habit is the first step on this journey. Are you striving for a healthier body, aiming to boost your confidence, or simply looking to have more energy for your daily activities? Whatever your motivation, it's essential to keep it in mind, as it will serve as your driving force.

Now, let's talk about the psychology of motivation. Human beings are wired to seek pleasure and avoid pain. So, make your core workouts enjoyable! Find activities that you genuinely love, whether it's dancing, hiking, or playing a sport. When you have fun, it won't feel like a chore, and you'll be more likely to stick with it.

But here's the secret sauce: accountability and the power of community. Surrounding yourself with like-minded individuals who share your fitness goals can be a game-changer. Join a local fitness class, join an online group, or grab a workout buddy. When you have people cheering you on and expecting you to show up, it becomes much more challenging to skip those core exercises.

Speaking of accountability, tracking your progress is vital. Keep a workout journal or use a fitness app to monitor your achievements. When you see your strength and endurance improve, it's not just physically rewarding; it's also a tremendous motivator.

Now, let's address the elephant in the room: time. We all lead busy lives, and it can be challenging to find the hours to dedicate to exercise. But here's the good news - you don't need hours! Short, effective core workouts can be as beneficial as long ones. Even just 15-20 minutes a day can make a significant difference over time.

Incorporate core exercises into your daily routine. Whether you're watching TV, waiting for dinner to cook, or brushing your teeth, seize those moments to sneak in some planks, leg raises, or bicycle crunches. These small, consistent efforts add up and become a part of your lifestyle.

Remember, it's not about perfection; it's about progress. Don't be discouraged by setbacks or missed workouts. Life happens, and that's okay. What's essential is that you get back on track, one step at a time. Consistency is the key to success in making core exercise a part of your lifestyle.

As you embark on this journey, you'll experience personal success. You'll feel stronger, more energized, and confident. This success will ripple into other areas of your life. You'll find that you're more disciplined, focused, and resilient in facing challenges. It's not just about a flat stomach; it's about developing a mindset of perseverance and determination.

Moreover, your personal success will inspire others. When friends, family, or coworkers see the positive changes in you, they'll be curious and motivated to follow in your footsteps. Your journey becomes a beacon of hope, showing that anyone can make core exercise a lifestyle.

Real people, just like you, are breaking free from the shackles of sedentary lifestyles and discovering the transformative power of core exercise. Their stories resonate because they mirror your own journey towards a healthier, more vibrant life.

Meet Jane, a busy mother of two, juggling a full-time job and family responsibilities. She used to dread feeling sluggish and tired all the time. One day, she decided to incorporate core exercises into her daily routine. Initially, it was tough, but she persevered. Soon enough, Jane felt stronger, her posture improved, and her energy soared. She wasn't just physically fitter; her mood lifted, and her stress levels plummeted.

Then there's Mike, a retiree who thought age had him cornered. His persistent back pain made everyday tasks a challenge. Mike embarked on a journey of core exercise. Slowly but surely, his pain eased, and he regained the agility of his youth. His newfound strength gave him confidence, and he found himself taking up hobbies he thought were long gone.

These stories are like beacons, shining light on the incredible transformation that core exercise can bring.

The Power of Core Exercise: A Life-Changer

Whether you're a college student or a grandparent, core exercises can be your lifestyle's cornerstone. They're not just about getting those abs of steel; they're about revitalizing your entire being. The journey begins with embracing your initial struggles and learning from them.

Imagine your core as the epicenter of your body's strength, stability, and vitality. When it's strong, you can conquer life's challenges with grace and resilience.

Let's dive into these incredible stories of transformation and discover the key core exercises that can make a difference in your life.

Jane's Journey to Renewed Vitality

Jane's tale of transformation is one we can all relate to. The hustle and bustle of daily life had left her feeling drained and disconnected from her own body. But Jane decided she deserved better.

She started with simple exercises like planks and Russian twists. At first, her core quivered, but she pressed on. Gradually, she noticed a change. Her posture improved, her back pain eased, and her stamina skyrocketed. No longer did she slump at her desk; she stood tall and confident.

What's more, the emotional and mental impact was astounding. Jane's newfound strength gave her a sense of empowerment. Her family noticed her increased positivity and zest for life. Core exercise became her daily ritual, a source of not just physical strength but emotional resilience.

Mike's Age-Defying Journey

Mike's story challenges the notion that age is an insurmountable barrier. His persistent back pain had made him feel trapped in an aging body. But Mike was determined to rewrite this narrative.

With the guidance of a fitness expert, he started incorporating exercises like leg raises and bridges into his daily routine. Initially, it wasn't easy, but Mike didn't give up. Gradually, he felt his back pain receding. His posture improved, and he regained the flexibility he thought he had lost forever.

More than just physical improvements, Mike's mental outlook underwent a complete transformation. He felt a renewed sense of purpose and confidence. With each core exercise, he defied the limitations of his age. He started hiking and playing golf again, hobbies he had almost abandoned.

Before and After: A Glimpse of Transformation

To add depth and authenticity, here are some before-and-after insights from our transformational heroes:

Jane's Before: "I felt exhausted and overwhelmed, lacking the energy to enjoy life."

Jane's After: "I'm full of energy, standing tall, and embracing every moment with enthusiasm."

Mike's Before: "Back pain had me trapped in a sedentary routine, feeling old beyond my years."

Mike's After: "I'm reclaiming my vitality, defying age, and enjoying my favorite activities again."

As you embark on your core exercise journey, remember that these transformations are not reserved for a select few. They're within your reach, waiting for you to take the first step.

Conclusion: Core Exercise as Your Lifestyle

Incorporating core exercise into your daily life is not just about aesthetics; it's about embracing vitality, strength, and resilience. Jane and Mike's stories – along with the core exercises they embraced – illustrate the power of a transformed core.

So, why wait? Start your own journey today. Your core holds the key to a healthier, happier, and more vibrant you. Embrace the struggle, celebrate the progress, and savor the transformation. You've got this!

Here's another book by Scott Hamrick that you might like

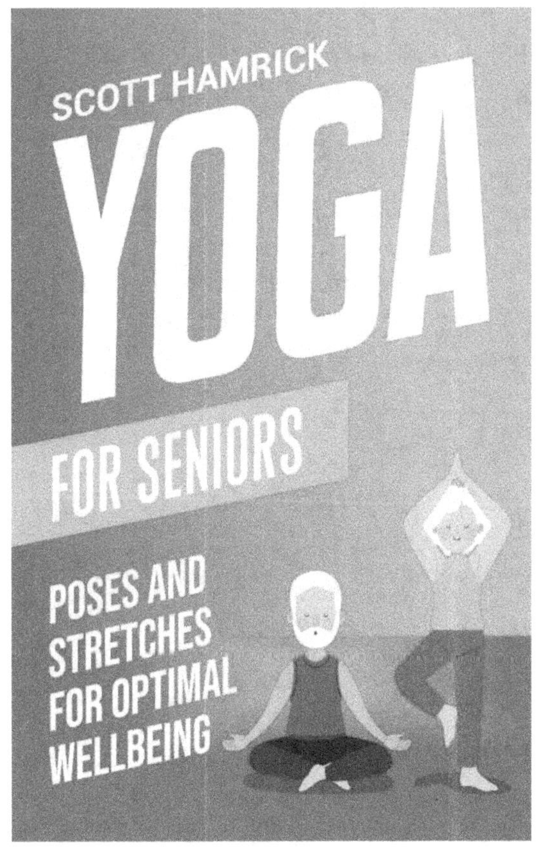

Free Bonuses from Scott Hamrick

Hi seniors!

My name is Scott Hamrick, and first off, I want to THANK YOU for reading my book.

Now you have a chance to join my exclusive "workout for seniors" email list so you can get the ebook below for free as well as the potential to get more ebooks for seniors for free! Simply click the link below to join.

P.S. Remember that it's 100% free to join the list.

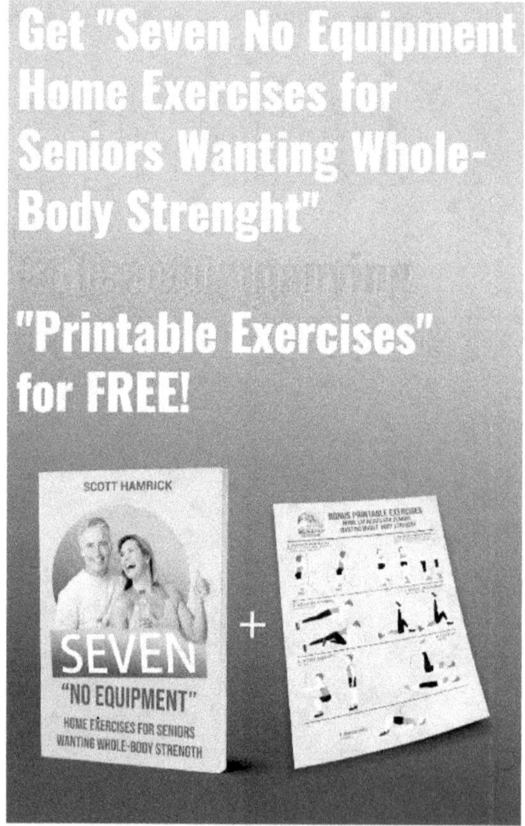

Access your free bonuses here
https://livetolearn.lpages.co/core-exercises-for-seniors-paperback/

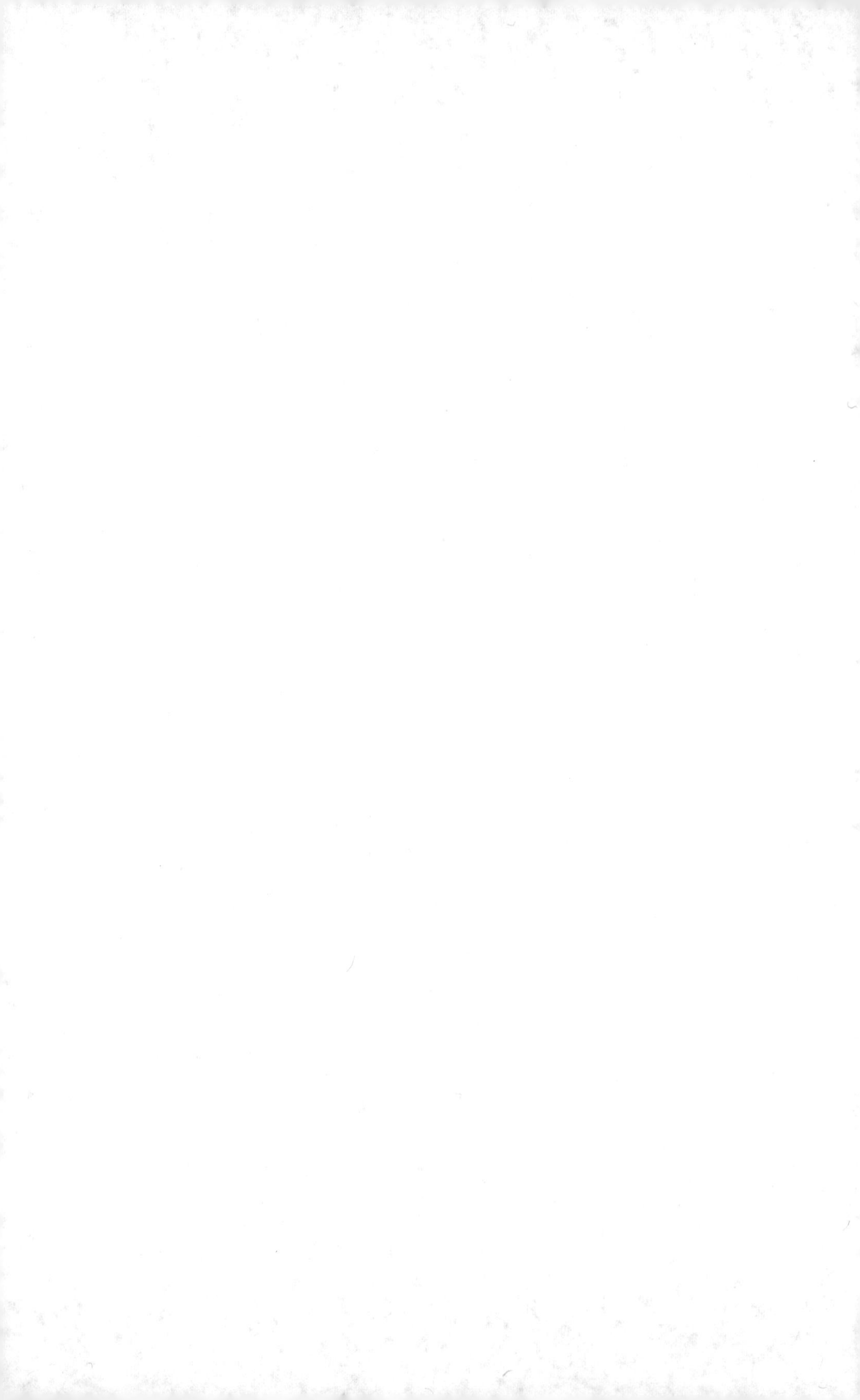